100 Questions & Answers About Lung Cancer

Karen Parles, MLS
Editor, LungCancerOnline

Joan H. Schiller, MD
Professor of Medicine, University of Wisconsin

JONES AND BARTLETT PUBLISHERS
Sudbury, Massachusetts
BOSTON   TORONTO   LONDON   SINGAPORE

World Headquarters
Jones and Bartlett
Publishers
40 Tall Pine Drive
Sudbury, MA 01776
info@jbpub.com
www.jbpub.com

Jones and Bartlett
Publishers Canada
2406 Nikanna Road
Mississauga, ON L5C
2W6
CANADA

Jones and Bartlett
Publishers International
Barb House, Barb Mews
London W6 7PA
UK

Library of Congress Cataloging-in-Publication Data
Parles, Karen.
    100 questions & answers about lung cancer / Karen Parles, Joan H. Schiller.
        p. cm.
Includes index.
    ISBN 0-7637-2376-2
1. Lungs–Cancer–Popular works. I. Title: One hundred questions and answers about lung cancer. II. Schiller, J. H. (Joan H.), 1954- III. Title.
    RC280.L8 P365 2003
    616.99'424–dc21

                                                                                    2002007066

Acquisitions Editor: Christopher Davis
Production Editor: Elizabeth Platt
Cover Design: Philip Regan
Manufacturing Buyer: Therese Bräuer
Composition: Northeast Compositors
Printing and Binding: Malloy Lithographing
Cover Printer: Malloy Lithographing

Printed in the United States of America

06 05 04 03 02 10 9 8 7 6 5 4 3 2

Contents

Part 1: The Basics   1

Questions 1–6 provide background information for understanding lung cancer, covering such topics as:

- What should I know about cancer cells?
- How do normal lungs function?
- Are there different types of lung cancer?
- What causes lung cancer?

Part 2: Diagnosis & Staging   11

Questions 7–17 describe the symptoms of lung cancer and discuss how lung cancer is diagnosed and staged:

- What are the symptoms of lung cancer?
- Which tests are performed to diagnose lung cancer?
- What are lymph nodes?
- What is staging, and why is it important?

Part 3: Coping with Your Diagnosis   23

Questions 18–30 address the medical, emotional, and practical aspects of coping with a lung cancer diagnosis:

- What is my prognosis? Can I survive lung cancer?
- Should I get a second opinion?
- How do I manage my emotions?
- What do caregivers need to know?
- What insurance and financial concerns do I need to address following a lung cancer diagnosis?

Part 4: Treatment   55

Questions 31–70 describe the types of treatments available for lung cancer (including surgery, chemotherapy, radiation, clinical trials, and complementary and alternative therapies) and address the challenges of evaluating treatment options.

- What does my surgeon mean when she says she "got it all"?
- What are the treatment options for my type and stage of lung cancer?
- How do I learn about clinical trials?
- What should I know about complementary and alternative therapies?

When I was asked by Karen Parles and Joan Schiller to write the Foreword to *100 Questions & Answers About Lung Cancer*, I was not only honored to say yes, but also pleased to see two people with so much experience writing a much-needed book. Lung cancer, the most common cause of cancer death in the United States, killing more people every year than breast, colon, and prostate cancers combined, is a neglected and under-reported disease. A media survey commissioned by Cancer Care in 2000, reviewing 600 news stories about cancer, confirmed what we already knew: that lung cancer receives far less coverage in print, broadcast, and online news than the three other major cancers. There are few celebrities, few events, few first-person stories, and little attention to progress in detection or treatment of lung cancer. Most coverage of lung cancer is directed to tobacco as its primary cause. Research dollars for lung cancer are limited, with less than $1000 spent per death, compared to $9000 per death for breast cancer or $3500 for prostate cancer.

I have spent my professional life of more than 25 years working in the field of cancer, and I am well aware that "competition" among diseases is not productive for patients, clinicians, or researchers. However, it's clearly time to focus on lung cancer and provide education, support, and increased research funding to this disease. Lung cancer remains the cancer that is stigmatized, with a "blame the victim" attitude. This perception, held by the lay public and many professionals, leads to isolation for people coping with this illness and frequently prevents them from understanding treatment options. It is crucial that people diagnosed with lung cancer know that they have the right to seek information, ask questions, and have a clear understanding of the choices available. A book such as this one gives the patient and family crucial information and support that they need to cope at a time of anxiety and confusion. Karen and Joan are leaders in their respective fields of patient advocacy and medical oncology, and the experience and knowledge that they bring provides an outstanding resource for anyone concerned about lung cancer. They represent just what we have been seeking for many years: experienced, knowledgeable individuals who are ready to speak out about lung cancer.

As Executive Director of Cancer Care, I have had the opportunity to develop support and education services for people with lung cancer, and I have participated in media programs focused on lung cancer awareness. Karen Parles and Joan Schiller are in the vanguard of committed advocates and professionals who want to seize this moment and add their articulate voices to the growing interest in lung cancer. *100 Questions & Answers About Lung Cancer* will be a cornerstone of our burgeoning efforts to have an impact on this difficult disease; it will enable patients and families to seek out the best treatment with the goal of the best possible outcome. Progress is being made in detection and treatment of lung cancer: we need to get that word out, and Karen and Joan are experts who are using their extensive experience to provide accurate information, support, and, importantly, hope to the tens of thousands of people coping with lung cancer.

With *100 Questions & Answers About Lung Cancer*, no one with lung cancer need be alone in the fight against the disease. Use it as an information source, seek support, ask questions: you have a wonderful resource available to you right here.

Diane Blum
Executive Director of Cancer Care
June 3, 2002

Janet M. Healy
Advocacy Program Manager
Alliance for Lung Cancer Advocacy, Support, and Education (ALCASE)

Since emerging as a significant disease just fifty years ago, lung cancer has grown to be a major public health challenge nationally and globally. But if you or someone you care about has lung cancer, its personal impact is most compelling. Complex decisions must be made quickly, and a sense of isolation, fear, and even guilt can complicate the process. Where to turn for information, the best medical care, and personal support? *100 Questions & Answers About Lung Cancer*, by authors personally familiar with the disease, responds to these and many more concerns.

When the Alliance for Lung Cancer Advocacy, Support, and Education (ALCASE) was founded in 1995, there were very few resources for people facing the disease. It's gratifying that in the last five years, more organizations have developed information and support services. Several good books-most recently this one-are now available to help people with lung cancer navigate the medical system and find many sources of personal support. The Internet has been an enormous influence, too. Now there are lung cancer web sites hosted by organizations and lung cancer survivors (including Karen Parles). There are search engines for finding clinical trials. There are even e-mail Listservs and message boards for lung cancer survivors and their families. These developments create a virtual community of people most directly involved with lung cancer. They also result in educated and outspoken patients and families who seek physicians willing to work with them. Knowledge is power, and people who make informed decisions are more effective advocates for themselves and others.

Since ALCASE began, there has been measurable progress in lung cancer prevention, early detection, and treatment research. Clinical trials for screening methods are underway nationally, as is research to prevent lung cancer from developing in people already at risk for it. The National Cancer Institute funds six special centers for lung cancer research around the country, and other top academic institutions are pursuing molecular and genetic research into the causes and treatment of lung cancer. Many of these projects seek to target lung cancer cells much more specifically than current chemotherapies and to customize treatment to particular tumor types. The future holds the prospect of drugs with less toxicity and fewer side effects, too. There are advances in mapping and delivering radiation therapy as well. In recent years, there has also been a noticeable shift toward maintaining good quality of life for people receiving treatment for lung cancer. This includes more attention by medical professionals to patients' fatigue, pain, appetite, and emotional well-being. At last, more lung cancer support groups are available and there is good telephone support offered by other organizations that complements ALCASE's Hotline and Phone Buddy programs.

But much more remains to be done. There is a noticeable lack of private foundations to promote more lung cancer research. With few early symptoms, no recommended early detection methods, and frequent misdiagnosis, people often find out they have lung cancer when it's already in later stages. This means grappling with urgent, complex decisions while coming to terms with fear and uncertainty. It also can mean that people with lung cancer have little time or energy to become more publicly involved in lung cancer issues. Lung cancer advocacy is still in its infancy, compared with other diseases. Many more people need to engage in effective activism locally and nationally. Part of this work means confronting the tobacco industry's continuing influence here and abroad. The myth persists that smoking is a "lifestyle choice" rather than behavior resulting from drug addiction. But even if all smoking stopped tomorrow, lung cancer would be with us for decades. Lung cancer is still considered a willingly self-inflicted disease, and this blame affects media coverage of lung cancer stories, hampers fundraising for research, and chills compassion for people with the disease. Change will come as more people realize that no one "deserves" lung cancer. The opportunity to speak out on these and many other issues awaits everyone who is involved with lung cancer-survivors, families, physicians, and patient advocates. Adding celebrity "star-power" to our cause will boost our impact.

How far have we come in changing the course of lung cancer? There is measurable progress, but we must do better as a nation and world. *100 Questions & Answers About Lung Cancer* is part of the progress. It can help guide you toward the answers you seek and encourage you to live with hope during your journey.

People diagnosed with lung cancer face extraordinary emotional, physical, and practical challenges. Although these challenges can seem overwhelming at times, they are not insurmountable. Living with lung cancer can be made easier with information, support, and hope. In this book, *100 Questions & Answers About Lung Cancer*, we give you the information and tools you need to cope with your diagnosis and put yourself in the best position to survive your disease. We help you to become an effective patient and take an active role in your care. We tell you how to find the best doctor, why multidisciplinary care is so important, and when second opinions can be valuable. Because the quality of your care can be compromised by poor communication, we stress the importance of clear and open communication among everyone involved in patient care—from patient and caregiver to doctors, nurses, and social workers. We discuss why the relationship between doctor and patient is fundamental to good medical care and offer ways that you can work to strengthen that relationship. We believe that lung cancer is a disease that affects more than just individuals—patients, family members, and caregivers all experience stress and have psychosocial and practical needs that require attention. Our intention is to elucidate these needs, identify potential sources of support, and encourage patients, caregivers, and loved ones to seek out support services. Finally, we feel that by educating yourself about lung cancer and its treatments, you will know which questions to ask your doctors and be equipped to make informed decisions about your care. *100 Questions & Answers About Lung Cancer* provides you with information to start you on your way, and identifies resources that will extend your knowledge beyond the pages of this book. We hope that you will find its contents useful.

During the course of Joan's work as a physician and Karen's experiences as a patient and advocate, we have been humbled and touched by the courage of patients and by the dedication of lung cancer professionals. It is both an honor and a privilege to count ourselves among the ranks of people who are fighting to eradicate the devastation brought about by lung cancer. For allowing us the opportunity to collaborate on this book, we are grateful to Christopher Davis, Executive Publisher for Medicine at Jones & Bartlett Publishers. We thank Elizabeth Platt for her editorial expertise, and for her patience and support. Karen thanks her parents and brother, Shirley, Howard, and David DeLong, who provided comments on the manuscript and support in everything else. To her doctors, Thomas J. Lynch and John C. Wain, she expresses her admiration for their outstanding contributions and tireless efforts on behalf of lung cancer patients and her profound gratitude for the compassionate care she receives from them. Karen dedicates this book to her husband, Jamie, and her children, Chris and Casey, who light up her days and give meaning to her life. Joan dedicates this book to the strength, courage, and dignity of the thousands of people diagnosed each year with lung cancer and their families. She continues to be amazed and inspired by the strength and love of the human spirit, as demonstrated daily by these individuals.

Karen Parles, MLS
Joan H. Schiller, MD

The Basics

What is cancer?

What should I know about cancer cells?

How do normal lungs function?

More ...

1. What is cancer?

Cancer is uncontrolled growth of **cells**—the billions upon billions upon billions of microscopic units that make up all the organs of our body. Cells are easily distinguished from each other: lung cells are very different in appearance and function from colon cells, which are very different from blood cells, and so forth. To understand what cancer is, you must first understand some of the properties of normal cells.

Cells

microscopic units that make up the organs of the body

Normal cells "do their own thing." For example, red blood cells carry oxygen throughout the body, stomach cells absorb nutrients, and white blood cells fight infections. Normal cells also stop growing and dividing when they get too old. In addition, normal cells often "self destruct" (undergo **apoptosis**) and die if they are injured.

Apoptosis

process by which normal cells die; often referred to as "programmed cell death"

Cancer cells differ from normal cells in a number of important ways. First, they are often unable to stop growing and dividing ("unregulated growth"). Second, cancer cells often stop "doing their thing." In fact, they often stop doing anything useful at all. For example, cancerous white blood cells often stop fighting infection, stomach cancer cells stop absorbing nutrients, and lung cancer cells are unable to absorb oxygen. Another property of cancer cells is that they do not die like normal cells do when they grow old; they are literally immortal. In addition, cancer cells often spread to other organs, a process called **metastasis**. They can metastasize either by invading a nearby organ or by entering into the bloodstream or lymphatic system and traveling through the body to invade distant organs. Sometimes the only thing that stops cancer cells from growing and spreading is that they run out of blood supply.

Metastasis

the spread of cancer from the initial cancer site to other parts of the body

A **tumor** is a mass of tissue formed by a new growth of cells. If a tumor stops growing by itself, and does not invade other tissues, it is considered **benign**. Examples include lipomas, which are soft, spongy, fatty tumors that form on the skin. Most tumors are **malignant**, which means they exhibit all the properties of cancer cells we've just mentioned.

2. What should I know about cancer cells?

One generalization is that most cancer cells have mutations in their **DNA**. DNA is the "brains" of the cell; it is composed of **chromosomes**. Each cell in the human body contains 46 chromosomes. These chromosomes are made up of thousands of smaller units called **genes**; each of these genes regulates a particular function. For example, certain genes control the color of your hair, others control how tall you grow, others control whether you produce insulin. If a gene is accidentally damaged, the change is called a **mutation**. It is not always clear as to what causes mutations. Some mutations are inherited, some may be due to diet, and others might be caused by exposure to environmental factors, such as radon, or cancer-causing chemicals (**carcinogens**). Nicotine in cigarette smoke contains hundreds of powerful carcinogens. Some mutations damage the gene or chromosome to the point where it causes the gene to stop working. This may result in the death of the cell, which is a relatively unusual cause of cancer. Cancer is usually due to the unregulated growth of cells, not their deaths.

Most mutations that cause cancer do so by causing the genes to work incorrectly. Incidentally, many cancer cells have similar mutations. Many of these mutations

Tumor

a mass of tissue formed by a new growth of cells

Benign

not cancerous; not life-threatening

Malignant

cancerous; cells that exhibit rapid, uncontrolled growth and can spread to other parts of the body

DNA (deoxyribonucleic acid)

the "brains" of a cell; DNA is composed of chromosomes

Chromosomes

strands of DNA and proteins in cell nucleus; carry units of heredity (genes)

Gene

unit of heredity that regulates a particular function; located on a specific place on a chromosome

Mutation

a damaged gene

Carcinogens

cancer-causing substances

The Basics

that cause cancer occur in genes that govern how cells grow or how cells die. After a normal gene is mutated, it is called either an **oncogene** or **tumor suppressor gene**. Oncogenes are genes that normally help cells grow; when they are mutated, they cannot shut off, and the cells cannot stop growing. Tumor suppressor genes are genes that normally make injured or mutated cells stop growing. If they become mutated, they usually stop functioning, thus allowing mutated cells to grow unabated.

We also know that **growth factors** can be important in the development of cancer. Growth factors are substances made by cancer cells or (sometimes) normal cells. Estrogen, for example, is a growth factor required for normal functions in breast and ovarian cells, but it can also cause some types of breast cancer cells to grow and divide. Some growth factors made by cancer cells tell other cells to proliferate. An example of this is vascular epithelial growth factor (VEGF), a growth factor made by cancer cells that stimulates growth of new blood vessels. This is one way that tumors encourage blood vessels to grow into them, which is another common characteristic of cancer: it often needs blood vessels to support its growth. New blood vessels rarely form in adults, except in certain circumstances such as wound healing or pregnancy. Blood vessels are necessary for a tumor to grow, as they deliver oxygen and nutrients to the tumor. They can also sometimes serve as a "highway" for tumor cells to travel as they spread throughout the body. Formation of new blood vessels is sometimes called **angiogenesis** (angio = blood; genesis = new; angiogenesis = formation of new blood vessels) or **neovascularization** (neo = new; vascularization

Oncogene

a mutated gene that can allow a cell to grow uncontrollably

Tumor suppressor gene

a gene that can block cancer from developing

Growth factors

substances that stimulate cells to grow

Angiogenesis

the formation of new blood vessels that allows tumors to grow

Neovascularization

angiogenesis; the formation of new blood vessels

= development of blood vessels; neovascularization = development of new blood vessels).

3. How do normal lungs function?

Lungs are necessary for breathing—that is, bringing oxygen into the body and getting rid of carbon dioxide. Oxygen is necessary for cells to make energy, and a by-product of the energy-producing process is carbon dioxide, which needs to be removed from the body. This critical oxygen–carbon dioxide exchange takes place in the lungs.

When we inhale air, it travels through the main breathing tube called the **trachea**, which divides into two tubes **(main stem bronchi)** in the area near the heart. One division goes to the right lung **(right main stem bronchus)** and the other to the left **(left main stem bronchus)**. From there, the bronchi divide into smaller and smaller segments until they eventually become so tiny and thin that they evolve into **alveoli**. Alveoli are the millions of microscopic air sacs through which oxygen diffuses into red blood cells in the blood to be taken everywhere in the body. In exchange, carbon dioxide carried by the red blood cells from the body diffuses into the alveoli; it is then expelled out of the body through the airways when we exhale.

Notice that each lung is divided into sections called lobes. The right lung has three lobes, but the left lung has only two to make room for the heart. The heart assists in the vital process of breathing by pumping blood to and from the lungs (Figure 1).

The Basics

Trachea

breathing tube (airway) leading from the larynx to the lungs

Main stem bronchi

the two main breathing tubes (right main stem bronchus and left main stem bronchus) that branch off the trachea

Main stem bronchus

see main stem bronchi

Alveoli

tiny air sacs that compose the lungs

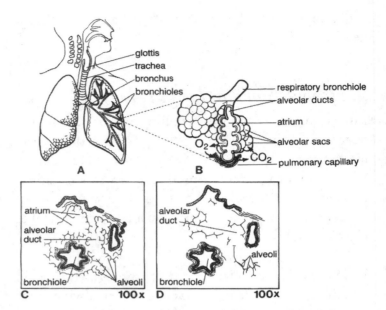

Figure 1   Internal structure of the lungs. A. Relationship of the lungs to the head and neck. B. External and internal appearance of a lung lobule, showing the atrium and alveolar sacs. C. Section of a lung, magnified 100 times. D. Section of a similar lung with emphysema. Note the decreased number of alveolar sacs and consequent diminishing in the gas exchange area of lung tissue. Reprinted from Anderson PD and Spitzer VM: *Human Anatomy and Physiology Coloring Workbook and Study Guide,* **Second Ed. Copyright © 1997, Jones and Bartlett Publishers, Inc.**

Squamous cell carcinoma

a type of non-small cell lung cancer

Adenocarcinoma

a type of non-small cell lung cancer; a malignant tumor that arises from glandular tissue

Large cell carcinoma

a type of non-small cell lung cancer

Small cell carcinoma

a type of lung cancer that differs in appearance and behavior from non-small cell lung cancers

4. Are there different types of lung cancer?

There are four different types of lung cancer: **squamous cell carcinoma, adenocarcinoma, large cell carcinoma,** and **small cell carcinoma.** These different types are distinguished by their appearance under the microscope. In the United States, adenocarcinoma is the most common, representing about 40% of all lung cancers. Three of these types (squamous cell carcinoma, adenocarcinoma, and large cell carcinoma) behave and are treated very similarly. They are sometimes collectively called **non-small cell lung cancer** (NSCLC), to distinguish them from **small cell lung cancer (SCLC)**, or small cell carcinoma.

Small cell lung cancer represents roughly 20–25% of all lung cancers. It differs from the three types of non-small cell lung cancer in several important ways: it tends to be more rapidly growing, cause symptoms quicker, and spread more rapidly. SCLC also tends to be more sensitive to chemotherapy and radiation therapy than NSCLC. For these reasons, treatment of SCLC is rarely surgery; rather, it is more commonly chemotherapy, sometimes with radiation therapy (see Question 55).

There is one sub-type of adenocarcinoma that bears mentioning: **bronchioloalveolar carcinoma** (BAC). BAC is a rare form lung cancer that represents only about 5% of all lung cancers, although there is reason to believe that the **incidence** of BAC is rising. BAC is unique in that it tends to spread diffusely throughout the alveoli (see Question 3), unlike the more typical lung cancer cells, which tend to "stick together" and form solid, discrete masses. The cause of BAC is less clear than for other forms of lung cancer. It tends to occur in younger, nonsmoking women. Of all the types of lung cancer, it is the one that may not be associated with smoking, although it is also found in smokers. BAC is similar to a disease found in sheep that is caused by a virus; scientists are trying to determine whether BAC is also caused by a virus, but at this point, the evidence is inconclusive. (For more information on BAC, see Question 64.)

The Basics

Non-small cell lung cancer (NSCLC)

a type of lung cancer that includes adenocarcinoma, squamous cell carcinoma, and large cell carcinoma

Small cell lung cancer (SCLC)

refers to small cell carcinoma, as opposed to non-small cell lung cancers (adenocarcinoma, squamous cell carcinoma, large cell carcinoma)

Bronchioloalveolar carcinoma (BAC)

a type of adenocarcinoma

Incidence

the number of new cases of a cancer (or any disease or event) in a defined population during a set period of time

5. What causes lung cancer?

Eighty-five to 90 percent of lung cancers are caused by carcinogens in nicotine that cause damage (mutations) to lung cells. People are usually exposed to nicotine in cigarette smoke by directly inhaling it while smoking; sometimes, people can develop lung cancer because they have inhaled large quantities of smoke from other smokers (**passive smoking**). Chronic exposure to asbestos, radon, and certain other environmental carcinogens can also cause lung cancer. When this occurs, it is invariably a result of long-term, occupational exposure. (See Questions 96–98 for information on lung cancer risk, screening, and prevention.)

Eighty-five to 90 percent of lung cancers are caused by carcinogens in nicotine.

Passive smoking

inhaling second-hand smoke

6. Who gets lung cancer? Is it common? Are the demographics changing?

Lung cancer is second only to prostate cancer in men and breast cancer in women in **incidence** (the number of new occurrences in a defined population during a set time period). Unfortunately, it is a very lethal disease; despite being second in incidence, it is nevertheless the leading cause of cancer death among both men and women. Lung cancer is responsible for more cancer-related deaths than breast cancer, colon cancer, and prostate cancer combined. Among racial and ethnic groups, lung cancer affects African-Americans disproportionately: African-Americans have the highest incidence and death rates of lung cancer.

Lung cancer is responsible for more cancer-related deaths than breast cancer, colon cancer, and prostate cancer combined.

Lung cancer is most commonly found in current or former smokers, usually in their early 60s. The incidence of lung cancer has been on the rise since smoking became popular in the 1920s and 1930s, but it began to rise rapidly around 1960, when the effects of the "cigarette boom" during the World War II years became evident. The death rate for lung cancer in men peaked in the late 1980s; however, it continues to rise in women. Many people do not realize that lung cancer is the leading cancer killer of both men and women. Of note, although stopping smoking significantly decreases the risk of lung cancer, approximately 50% of all lung cancers occur in former smokers.

Diagnosis and Staging

What are the symptoms of lung cancer?

How is lung cancer diagnosed?

What is staging and why is it important?

More ...

7. What are the symptoms of lung cancer?

The primary symptoms of lung cancer depend upon its location. If a cancer occurs near the center of the chest, for example, it often presses on a major airway or blood vessel. In these cases, common symptoms include cough (including blood-tinged **sputum**) and shortness of breath. If the tumor blocks or obstructs a major airway, bacteria and secretions can back up behind the obstruction, resulting in a "post-obstructive" **pneumonia**.

Other structures near the center of the chest are sometimes affected by lung cancer. Rarely, the recurrent laryngeal nerve may be involved. The recurrent laryngeal nerve goes from the brain to the vocal cords. Because of the way humans develop as fetuses, this nerve does not make a direct path from the brain to the vocal cord, as one might expect. Instead, it travels down to the chest and then back up again, swinging by the major vessels leading in and out of the heart. If the tumor happens to impinge upon this nerve, hoarseness can result. Similarly, if the tumor happens to impinge upon the **esophagus**, the "feeding tube" that leads from the mouth to the stomach, patients can experience problems with choking or swallowing. If the tumor actually presses on one of the great vessels leading into the heart, such as the superior vena cava, the blood sometimes cannot flow easily into the heart and instead backs up into the neck, shoulders, and arms (**superior vena cava syndrome**). In this case, patients can experience swelling of these areas.

If the tumor arises farther out in the lung near the chest wall, patients can experience pain. Indeed, this is often the only time patients experience pain from lung

Sputum

mucous and other secretions produced by the lungs

Pneumonia

an inflammatory infection of the lung

Esophagus

the tube through which food travels from the mouth to the stomach

Superior vena cava syndrome (SVCS)

a collection of symptoms that may include swelling in the neck, shoulders, and arms caused by a lung tumor pressing on the SVC, one of the large vessels leading into the heart cancer, as this is really the only area of the lung that has nerve endings. The middle of the lung in the area near the heart does not have many nerve endings, so tumors that arise in these areas rarely cause pain. This is one of the reasons why lung cancer can grow unnoticed for a long period of time: it is painless unless the chest wall is involved.

Tumors arising near the chest wall can also cause a **pleural effusion** (see Question 76). A pleural effusion is an accumulation of fluid between the outside of the lung and the inside of the chest wall. This fluid can cause both pain and shortness of breath.

Pleural effusion
accumulation of fluid between the outside of the lung and the inside of the chest wall

If the tumor occurs near the top of the lung (**Pancoast tumor** or **superior sulcus tumor**), it may grow into some of the nerves leaving the spinal cord and traveling down through the armpit and into the arm. In this case, it can cause shoulder pain or weakness, or an unusual constellation of symptoms consisting of a droopy eyelid, dry eyes, and lack of sweating on the face.

Pancoast tumor (superior sulcus tumor)
a tumor occurring near the top of the lungs that may cause shoulder pain or weakness, or a group of symptoms including a droopy eyelid, dry eyes, and lack of sweating on the face.

If the tumor metastasizes, the symptoms will be related to the area of the body to which it has spread. For example, if the cancer spreads to the bone, it may cause pain in the back, hip, leg, or arm. If it spreads to the brain, it can cause headaches, nausea, or signs and symptoms similar to a stroke. These symptoms are not unique to metastatic lung cancer—any cancer that spreads to these organs will cause similar symptoms.

The most frequent symptoms of cancer, however, are fatigue, weakness, loss of appetite, and weight loss. These symptoms usually indicate that the cancer is advanced.

The most frequent symptoms of cancer are fatigue, weakness, loss of appetite, and weight loss.

8. Are there other symptoms associated with lung cancer?

Sometimes tumors can cause **paraneoplastic** symptoms. Paraneoplastic symptoms occur at a site not directly involved with the tumor. Presumably, the tumor must be making some type of hormone to affect these distant sites. Common paraneoplastic syndromes include **electrolyte** abnormalities (such as calcium and sodium imbalances), **neuropathy** (numbness and tingling of the hands and feet), and **clubbing** of the fingers. Clubbing is a manifestation of many different types of lung problems (not only lung cancer) that causes the nails on the fingers to bulge out somewhat. The cause of this effect is not known.

9. How is lung cancer diagnosed?

The diagnosis of lung cancer frequently is made when a patient goes to his or her primary care physician with complaints consistent with a bronchitis or pneumonia. Very often, these symptoms include cough, shortness of breath, and low-grade fevers. Because these symptoms are so common, they are often treated with antibiotics without taking a chest **x-ray**. If the symptoms do not resolve, however, a chest x-ray is eventually obtained, revealing some type of mass in the chest. The x-ray is frequently followed by a chest **CT scan** to provide more accurate details of the lungs and chest. This, in turn, often results in a **biopsy** (sampling of tissue), which is required for the diagnosis for any type of cancer. (CT scan and biopsy are discussed further in Question 10.)

Paraneoplastic symptoms

symptoms that result from substances released by cancer cells and that occur at a site not directly involved with the tumor

Electrolytes

acids, bases, and salts essential for maintaining life; electrolyte abnormalities are imbalances of salts or chemicals in the blood

Neuropathy

numbness and tingling of the hands and feet

Clubbing

a condition in which the nails on the fingers bulge out, a symptom of many different types of lung problems.

X-ray

high-energy radiation used to image the body

CT scan (computed tomography)

computerized series of x-rays that create a detailed cross-sectional image of the body

It is also not uncommon for lung cancer to be discovered accidentally on a chest x-ray or a CT scan taken for an unrelated condition. Currently, there is no approved screening test for lung cancer in **asymptomatic** (symptom-free) individuals who may be at risk for lung cancer (see Question 97).

10. Which tests are performed to diagnose lung cancer?

A computed tomography or CT scan (sometimes called a CAT scan) is the most helpful imaging test for characterizing an abnormality in the lung. CT scans are a series of x-rays in which the body is "sliced up" like a pack of Lifesavers. Each one of the slices is then called up on a computer screen to give a cross-sectional image of the chest. A CT scan offers considerably more detail than a regular chest x-ray. To help the radiologist distinguish between blood vessels and tumors on CT scans, a dye called CT or IV contrast is sometimes injected into the vein to make the blood vessels more pronounced.

Once a suspicious abnormality is detected on a CT scan, the patient needs a biopsy to obtain a definitive diagnosis. There are several ways of doing this. These include:

1. Bronchoscopy. A **bronchoscopy** is a procedure in which a lung doctor (**pulmonologist**) inserts a flexible tube called a **bronchoscope** through the nose down into the lungs. The bronchoscope, which has fiber optic lighting inside, has several purposes. It

---

Biopsy

removal of tissue or fluid sample for microscopic examination

---

It is not uncommon for lung cancer to be discovered accidentally on a chest x-ray or a CT scan taken for an unrelated condition.

Asymptomatic

without symptoms

Bronchoscopy

a procedure that involves inserting a flexible tube (bronchoscope) through the nose down into the lungs. Needles can be inserted through the bronchoscope to obtain biopsy samples.

Pulmonologist

a physician who specializes in the diagnosis and treatment of lung diseases

Bronchoscope

see Bronchoscopy

can serve as a "periscope," allowing the pulmonologist to see into the airways. Additionally, needles can be inserted through the bronchoscope to obtain biopsies. Although bronchoscopy is a commonly used diagnostic test, it does have several disadvantages. First, the pulmonologist usually cannot get the tube into the distant areas of the lung—the airways near the chest wall are too small to permit passing of the bronchoscope. Therefore, the use of this test is limited to inspection of the major bronchi, or airways. Second, if the cancer itself is not actually growing in the airway, it can be difficult for the pulmonologist to get a biopsy, because he or she cannot actually see the tumor.

Transthoracic (percutaneous) biopsy

a biopsy obtained by inserting a needle through the skin and chest wall into the tumor

2. **Transthoracic** or **percutaneous biopsy**. Specialized doctors, called **interventional radiologists**, can sometimes insert a needle through the skin and chest wall into the tumor in order to obtain tissue for a biopsy. This procedure usually does not require a hospital stay (outpatient procedure).

Interventional radiologist

a radiologist who uses x-rays and other imaging techniques to perform minimally invasive medical procedures

3. **Surgery.** Sometimes, the abnormality seen on chest x-ray or CT scan cannot be easily biopsied by either a bronchoscopy or a transthoracic biopsy. In this case, patients may have to undergo surgery. The surgeon can do several different procedures to make the diagnosis. These include:

Mediastinoscopy

a surgical procedure by which lymph nodes can be removed for microscopic examination

• **Mediastinoscopy.** This procedure involves making a small incision above the collarbone or between the spaces of the first and second or second and third ribs. The surgeon then inserts a special tube through this incision into the mediastinum. Again, this tube has two functions: it allows the surgeon to see the lymph nodes near the heart, and it also allows the surgeon to biopsy them. A mediastinoscopy is sometimes done not only to make the diagnosis of cancer, but also to help "stage" the patient (see Question 13).

- **Mini-thoracotomy** or **video-assisted thoracoscopic surgery (VATS).** Both of these procedures involve making an incision someplace on the outside of the chest and inserting a tube into the space between the chest wall and the lung. This allows a surgeon to see the outside of the lung and to biopsy any suspicious areas.

Mini-thoracotomy
a type of minimally invasive chest surgery

11. How will I learn about the results of my biopsy? What information will be in the pathology report, and what will it mean for me?

It typically takes two to three days before the biopsy results become available. We strongly suggest that you schedule an appointment with your doctor to receive the results and discuss your **prognosis** and treatment options. There is nothing worse than getting bad news over the phone, when the doctor may not have much time to talk to you.

There is nothing worse than getting bad news over the phone.

Prognosis
predicted outcome; likelihood of survival

A specialized doctor called a **pathologist** looks at the biopsy samples under the microscope. He or she tries to answer the following critical questions:

Pathologist
a physician trained to examine and evaluate cells and tissue.

- *Is it cancer?* The pathologist determines this by judging how "normal" the cells look. Part of the definition of cancer is that normal cells become very abnormal and no longer look or function like the type of cells they are supposed to be. The question as to whether something is cancerous is not always straightforward. Typically, normal cells from different parts of our body look very different microscopically and are easy to tell apart—blood cells look very different from muscle cells, for example. In many tumors, the cells are so wildly abnormal looking that one cannot tell where they originated from or from what part of the body they were taken. However, in some cases the cells look only "very abnormal," and in others, "somewhat abnormal." Pathologists use the term **grade** or **differentiation** to describe the degree of abnormality of the appearance of the cells. Although the grade of a tumor is important in other types of cancer, in lung cancer it is often not even reported.

- *If it is cancer, what kind is it?* As discussed in Question 4, there are different types of lung cancer. Although the pathologist typically will call it one of the four major types (adenocarcinoma, squamous cell carcinoma, large cell carcinoma, or small cell carcinoma) based on its appearance microscopically, the most important distinction is whether it is small cell lung cancer or not.

Pathologists classify tumors into different **histological** types based upon the characteristics or patterns some tumors make. For example, adenocarcinomas often look like glands; large cell carcinomas contain—you guessed it—large cancer cells; and small cell cancers contain small cancer cells. One reason that pathologists classify tumors into one of these histologies (tissue types) is to help determine from where the cancer arose. As it turns out, many adult cancers that start in different parts of the body can also look glandular. For example, breast cancer, colon cancer, and prostate cancers are also adenocarcinomas.

Grade

a term used to describe the degree to which tumor tissue resembles normal tissue

Differentiation

grade; the degree to which tumor tissue resembles normal tissue

Histology/ histological

tissue type; assessment of cellular features by microscopic evaluation

- *If it is cancer, where did it come from?* If a tumor starts in the lung, it is called lung cancer. However, other cancers commonly spread to the lungs. If a tumor starts elsewhere in the body, say, the breast, and spreads to the lung, it is still called breast cancer. If a lung cancer spreads to the liver, for example, it is still called lung cancer. This is because in general, cancers typically behave like the cancer in its place of origin—breast cancer that has metastasized to the lung still tends to respond to breast cancer chemotherapy better than lung cancer chemotherapy, and tends to grow and behave similarly to breast cancer elsewhere in the body.

12. What are lymph nodes?

Lymph nodes are small collections of white blood cells scattered throughout the body. White blood cells not only flow through the bloodstream, they also flow through a second type of vascular system in our bodies called the **lymphatic system**. Unlike the other organs in our body, of which everyone has the same number (e.g., we all have two lungs, one liver, one heart), there are hundreds of different lymph nodes, and everyone has a different number of them.

Lymph nodes are important because sometimes cancer can spread through the lymphatic system. If the lymph nodes that your surgeon removes contain cancer, this implies that since your lung cancer got that far, it may also have escaped out of the lymph nodes and spread elsewhere in your body.

Lymph node

small collections of white blood cells scattered throughout the body

Lymphatic system

a vascular system that contains lymph nodes; cancer can spread through the lymphatic system.

Sometimes cancer can spread through the lymphatic system.

13. What is staging, and why is it important?

Staging a tumor involves determining how far a cancer has spread. This is useful for several reasons:

- It allows physicians to have a common "language" in describing a patient's tumor. Thus, when a surgeon tells an oncologist that a patient has Stage IIIA disease, the oncologist immediately has some idea as to the extent of the patient's disease.
- It is an important prognostic indicator. Patients with Stage I disease, for example, typically do much better than do patients with Stage IV disease.
- It is very useful for determining therapy. The type of treatment that is recommended—surgery, radiotherapy, chemotherapy, or any combination of these—will depend upon the extent of the disease and how far it has spread (i.e., the stage).

14. What are the staging guidelines for NSCLC?

The staging of cancer is classically dependent upon three criteria: the size and location of the tumor (**T** or tumor status); whether any lymph nodes are involved (**N** or nodal status); and whether the cancer has spread further than the lymph nodes (**M** or metastatic status). These three criteria (T, N, and M) are further subdivided. For example, if no lymph nodes contain tumor, this is called N0; if the local, or **hilar**, lymph nodes contain tumor, this is called N1; and if the lymph nodes between the lung and the heart, or **mediastinal** lymph nodes, contain tumor, this is typically called N2. N3 disease involves the lymph nodes in the other side of the chest, or in the area above the collar bone.

Table 1   Lung cancer staging based upon the TNM staging criteria

Stage I	Tumors that are small and do not have any lymph node involvement
Stage II	Tumors that have spread to the local (hilar) lymph nodes, OR tumors abutting the chest wall without lymph node involvement
Stage III	Tumors that are "locally advanced" but do not appear to have metastasized to distant organs
Stage IIIA	Tumors that are large and bulky but are still surgically **resectable** (i.e., the surgeon is technically able to take the tumor out), OR tumors that have spread to the mediastinal lymph nodes
Stage IIIB	Tumors that have not yet metastasized, but that are too large to resect or that are located such that the surgeon would be unable to resect them safely. Typical examples are tumors that have invaded the heart, one of the large blood vessels leading into or out of the heart, or one of the major airways. Also, patients with pleural effusion (see Question 76) and N3 lymph node involvement are classified as having Stage IIIB disease.
Stage IV	Tumors that have spread to other organs (**metastatic**)

Resectable

able to be surgically removed (resected)

Metastatic

tumors that have spread to other organs

Oncologists use a complicated system, based upon the TNM staging, determine the overall stage. A simplified summary is provided in Table 1.

15. What are the staging guidelines for SCLC?

Because SCLC tends to metastasize early, oncologists typically do not go into the formal "TNM" staging classification noted above. Instead, they typically divide SCLC into "limited stage" or "extensive stage" disease, in which limited stage is defined as cancer confined to one side of the chest, and extensive stage is defined as cancer that has spread outside the side of the chest from which it arose.

16. What are the common metastatic sites for lung cancer?

The most common metastatic sites for lung cancer are elsewhere in the lungs, the liver, the adrenal glands, the bones, and the brain.

17. Which tests and procedures are used to detect whether my lung cancer has spread beyond my chest?

Your oncologist may order a series of tests to determine whether the cancer has spread to one of the sites mentioned above. These might include a **bone scan** (an imaging test in which a radionuclear substance is injected into the veins and taken up by the bones in areas of potential metastatic disease), a head or abdominal CT scan, or a PET scan. **PET (positron emission tomography)** is a nuclear medicine scan that measures metabolism. Because cancer cells grow faster than normal cells, they presumably metabolize nutrients faster, a difference that can be picked up on a PET scan. A PET scan can help to determine whether abnormalities seen on CT are cancerous. However, your doctor is likely to order these tests only if there is some reason to suspect that the cancer has spread to these areas, such as laboratory test abnormalities or symptoms related to those organs (e.g., bone metastases may cause pain, brain metastases may cause signs or symptoms similar to a stroke, etc.).

Bone scan

an imaging test in which a radionuclear substance is injected into the veins and taken up by the bones in areas of potential metastatic disease

PET scan (positron emission tomography)

a nuclear medicine imaging test that measures metabolism; can differentiate between healthy and abnormal tissue

Coping With Your Diagnosis

What is my prognosis? Can I survive
lung cancer?

How do I manage my emotions?

Who treats lung cancer? What is
multidisciplinary care?

More . . .

Medical Aspects

18. What is my prognosis? Can I survive lung cancer?

It is natural to worry about what a lung cancer diagnosis will mean for you and your family and to wonder whether you will die from your cancer. Most patients want to know their prognosis so that they can plan for the future and prepare for what lies ahead. Your prognosis is a prediction of how well you will do and how long you will live. It is influenced by many factors, including the type of lung cancer you have, how far your cancer has spread, how aggressive your tumor is, your age, and your general health. The treatment you receive may affect your prognosis, and your prognosis may change over time. The best person to discuss your prognosis with is your doctor.

It is important to remember that your prognosis is only an educated guess.

To arrive at your prognosis, your doctor will take into consideration the lung cancer statistics, his or her experience with other lung cancer patients, and what he or she knows about your individual characteristics. It is important to remember that your prognosis is only an educated guess and that it is impossible for anyone, even your doctor, to predict your future with certainty.

Survival statistics for lung cancer may not be accurate for you.

You may become familiar with the survival statistics for lung cancer through discussions with your doctor or from other sources. For lung cancer patients, survival rates are not encouraging, and it can be overwhelming to learn about them. It is helpful to understand why these statistics may not be accurate for you. Survival statistics, like those compiled by the American Cancer Society, usually measure the 5-year survival of a group of patients with similar characteristics. They are population "averages" and do not represent the prognosis for any given individual. Your unique characteristics will cause your prognosis to differ from the population average. You should also be aware that the survival statistics reflect the outcomes of patients who were treated with older therapies. They don't take into account the newer, more effective treatments that are available today, or the promising treatments that will be available in the near future.

Although it makes sense to plan for every eventuality when you are facing a potentially deadly disease, you should not allow statistics, or a bleak prediction by your doctor, to dictate your future. There are patients who have survived every stage of lung cancer and patients who have outlived their doctors' predictions. Your prognosis provides a perspective, but it is not etched in stone. Try to focus your thoughts on the tens of thousands of people who have survived lung cancer. There is no reason why you can't be one of them.

Having said all that, however, while it is good to "hope for the best," you should also "prepare for the worst." Now is a good time to assess your personal, financial, and legal affairs (see Questions 29 and 95). Working on these issues while you are undergoing treatment in no way means you are "giving up." It may, however, relieve you of other worries down the road.

Although it is good to "hope for the best," you should also "prepare for the worst."

19. Who treats lung cancer? What is multidisciplinary care?

Lung cancer is a complex disease, and its treatment frequently involves some combination of surgery, chemotherapy, and radiation. You likely will see more than one specialist for your lung cancer care, including medical oncologists, thoracic surgeons, radiation oncologists, and pulmonologists. Ideally, these lung cancer doctors work together in a multidisciplinary clinic or other setting where they can easily consult with each other and reach a consensus about your treatment options. This multidisciplinary approach not only offers you high-quality care but also has practical advantages that may include fewer trips to the doctor, less time from diagnosis to start of treatment, and more efficient coordination of treatment logistics. Multidisciplinary care is commonly offered in cancer centers and in larger treatment centers such as university hospitals, but it is beginning to be implemented in some community hospitals as well.

Each lung cancer specialist you see is a member of your treatment team, but one doctor (usually the medical oncologist) will have primary responsibility for managing and directing your care. There are also a number of other doctors, along with support staff, who will be involved in your care. It is helpful to understand what each of these healthcare professionals does, and what role he or she plays in your care.

- **Medical oncologist:** a physician who performs comprehensive management of cancer patients throughout all phases of care. Medical oncologists specialize in treating cancer with medicine, using systemic treatments such as chemotherapy.
- **Thoracic surgeon:** a physician who specializes in performing chest surgery. A thoracic surgeon may have performed the tumor biopsy that resulted in your lung cancer diagnosis. Some thoracic surgeons

have received additional training in cancer surgery and are considered surgical oncologists.

- **Radiation oncologist:** a physician who specializes in treating cancer with radiation.
- **Pulmonologist:** a physician who specializes in the diagnosis and treatment of lung diseases. A pulmonologist may have diagnosed your lung cancer. You may also see a pulmonologist if you have ongoing respiratory issues related to your lung cancer, or underlying conditions such as **chronic obstructive pulmonary disease (COPD)**.

Other specialists or support staff:

- **Pathologist:** a physician trained to examine and evaluate cells and tissue. The pathologist evaluates your biopsy tissue and furnishes a biopsy report to your oncologist or surgeon.
- **Oncology nurse:** a specialized nurse trained to provide care to cancer patients, including administering chemotherapy and monitoring side effects.
- **Psychiatrist:** a physician who specializes in treating people for depression, anxiety, and other psychological illness. Psychiatrists provide psychotherapy and can also prescribe medication.
- **Psychologist:** a person trained in psychology who can provide psychotherapy.
- **Oncology social worker:** a social worker trained to provide counseling and practical assistance to cancer patients. Social workers can help you locate services such as transportation, support groups, and home care. They can also provide assistance with insurance and financial issues.

Chronic obstructive pulmonary disease (COPD)

chronic bronchitis or emphysema

- **Rehabilitation specialist:** a person trained to help patients recover from physical changes brought about by cancer or cancer treatment. Respiratory therapists help lung cancer patients to maximize their breathing capacity and learn to cope with breathlessness. Physical therapists can help patients recover range of motion and strength following lung cancer surgery.
- **Nutritionist** or **dietician:** a person trained to provide nutritional or dietary counseling. Lung cancer patients may experience weight loss as a result of their cancer or its treatment (see Question 82). Treatment side effects, such as nausea from chemotherapy or heartburn from radiation, can negatively affect appetite. Nutritional or dietary counseling services can help patients to increase appetite and gain weight.
- **Palliative care specialist:** a physician trained in cancer pain management.

20. How do I find the best doctors to treat my lung cancer? Does the hospital make any difference in my care?

There are resources you can turn to, and questions you can ask, to help you decide on the right doctor for you.

One of your primary responsibilities as a lung cancer patient is to be sure that you are getting the best care possible, starting with your choice of doctors. Although it is often difficult for patients to assess the quality of doctors and treatment centers, there are resources you can turn to, and questions you can ask, to help you decide on the right doctor for you.

The first step in finding a doctor or treatment center is to get a recommendation from a reliable source. Your primary care physician, or another doctor, can refer you to the best lung cancer specialists in your area. Other lung cancer patients are also good sources, as is the Alliance for Lung Cancer Advocacy, Support, and Education (ALCASE). If you cannot get a recommendation for a specific lung cancer specialist, you can contact the nearest cancer center or university hospital and ask for the names of their oncologists who specialize in lung cancer. The leading cancer centers are identified by the National Cancer Institute as NCI-designated cancer centers. The American College of Surgeons' Commission on Cancer also identifies hospitals with strong cancer programs. (For further information on these resources, and on others that will help you to locate doctors and cancer treatment centers, see Question 100.)

After you have the name of a doctor, you need to evaluate whether this person is a quality physician. Equally important, you need to decide whether you are comfortable with this person and whether the two of you will be able to communicate well with each other as you face the difficult decisions that lie ahead. Some things to consider:

• **Clinical experience.** It is critical to find out whether a physician has extensive experience with lung cancer patients. Oncologists treat patients with all types of cancers, but ideally you want to find an oncologist who specializes in lung cancer. This type of oncologist is referred to as a thoracic (or lung) oncologist and may be found at major cancer centers. Similarly, if you are seeking a surgeon, you want to find a thoracic or cardiothoracic surgeon who specializes in chest surgery, and not a general surgeon who performs all types of surgeries. Studies have shown that mortality is lower for lung cancer surgery when the surgery is performed by a thoracic surgeon. You should ask any prospective oncologist or surgeon what percentage of his or her practice is lung cancer patients.

- **Hospital affiliation.** It is important to consider your doctor's hospital affiliation. Cancer centers and university hospitals conduct research and provide access to the newest treatments and to **clinical trials** (see Questions 57 and 58). Patients are more likely to receive multidisciplinary care in these institutions and benefit from the collective expertise of multiple specialists. Patients who undergo surgery for lung cancer at hospitals that perform a large volume of lung surgery are likely to survive longer than patients who have similar surgery at hospitals with a low volume of lung cancer procedures.

  You should be aware, however, that cancer centers and university hospitals tend to be larger than community hospitals and often have residents (doctors in training) or medical students who see patients with the medical oncologist. This may seem more impersonal, especially at the beginning, but most people get used to these differences. Hospital affiliation should be a major factor in deciding who your physician will be.

- **Credentials.** Basic professional information for licensed U.S. physicians is available through the American Medical Association's Physician Select

Clinical trials

research studies involving people that test the safety and effectiveness of new treatments web site, *www.ama-assn.org/aps/amahg.htm*. Each listing offers information on the physician's medical school, residency and fellowship training, board certification, and office location. Board certification ensures proficiency in a specified area, such as medical oncology, radiation oncology, or thoracic surgery. Residency or fellowship training at a major cancer center can be a plus.

Other factors to consider:

- **Is the doctor covered by your insurance plan?** Financial constraints are a reality, and insurance is a limiting factor when selecting a doctor. There may be overriding reasons for consulting a specialist (or getting a second opinion) outside an insurance plan, but your primary lung cancer doctor needs to be covered by your policy unless cost is not an issue for you.
- **Distance.** Certain types of treatment (e.g., chemotherapy and radiation) require multiple trips to the doctor or hospital. For some people, distance from the doctor will be a significant issue. Ask the hospital social worker about transportation alternatives or possibilities for inexpensive lodging. If you really like the doctor but are worried about the distance you will have to travel, particularly if you are feeling tired or sick, ask whether the oncologist and your primary doctor would be willing to work together. Some doctors feel very comfortable with this type of arrangement, while others do not.
- **Alternative medicine**. If you are interested in alternative medicine, you should address this issue during your first visit. It is crucial that both you and your doctor are comfortable discussing alternative medicine issues, and that you are open with your

doctor about any use of alternative medicine (see Questions 61 and 62).

Because you are choosing a doctor who will be helping you to face life and death issues, the doctor's bedside manner, and your personal connection with him or her, are things to consider seriously. Trust and rapport are central to a strong doctor–patient relationship and should be given full consideration. Questions to ask yourself are:

- Does the doctor communicate in a clear and understandable manner? Is he or she willing to answer my questions? Is he or she a good listener?
- Does the doctor appear knowledgeable? Does the doctor inspire confidence?
- Does the doctor seem compassionate, caring, trustworthy?
- Did the doctor ask about me and my family—is he or she looking beyond my lung cancer?

After your appointment or consultation, you should have a positive feeling that you and your doctor can work together as partners. If you are not comfortable with the first doctor you visit, you should not hesitate to look for another one.

If you are not comfortable with the first doctor you visit, you should not hesitate to look for another one.

On the other hand, you should remember that doctors are people, too. Although every patient would like to have a doctor who is a world-class, internationally-known researcher with lots of time to spend with individual patients and a charismatic bedside manner, this isn't always going to be possible. The bottom line is that you need to feel comfortable that your doctor knows what he or she is doing, is interested in you as an individual, and is willing to talk to you and answer your questions.

21. Should I get a second opinion? What is a second pathology opinion?

The quality of your medical care is a critical factor in determining your chances for survival. A second opinion is an effective way to be sure you are getting the best possible care and, at the same time, to gain peace of mind that you have explored all of your options. There are certain cases when a second opinion is particularly important:

- If you have been told that you are not a candidate for surgery but have reason to think you might be, you should seek another opinion from a thoracic surgeon. Surgery offers the best chance for a cure from lung cancer, and concepts regarding who is an appropriate surgical candidate are changing. Some patients become candidates for surgery after chemotherapy and/or radiation are used to shrink their tumors.
- If your doctor tells you that there is no treatment available for you, don't give up. It is rarely the case that there are no treatment options. A second opinion provides a different perspective and may bring additional choices for treatment.
- If your doctor is associated with a small community hospital, it is a good idea to get a second opinion at a major cancer center or university hospital where research is performed, where the doctors may be more aware of the newest treatments, and where there may be additional clinical trial options for you.

- If you are uncomfortable with your doctor or have doubts about her recommendations for your care, you should look for another doctor. It is impossible to have a productive doctor-patient relationship if you do not have confidence and trust in your doctor.
- If there is a question about your diagnosis (your tumor type), you should get a second pathology opinion (see Question 22). Errors in pathology are unusual but can occur. Your prognosis and treatment plan are determined by your pathological diagnosis, a diagnosis made by a pathologist after examining your biopsy tissue. It is essential that your diagnosis is accurate.

Even when there is no compelling dilemma to resolve, a second opinion is still advisable. It can offer new options, confirm recommendations, or bring to light substandard care. If you get a conflicting second opinion, you can resolve issues by seeking a third opinion or by asking your primary care doctor (or another doctor) for guidance. Before seeking a second opinion, however, you should consider the potential downsides. The process of obtaining a second opinion can be emotionally draining, and will consume time and energy that you may not have. It can create confusion and delay treatment. You need to decide whether these negatives are offset by the potential long-term benefits of getting a second opinion.

Some patients worry that they will offend their doctor if they seek a second opinion. Keep in mind that you are entitled to seek a second opinion. Doctors are professionals who understand that patients will be seeking additional opinions or consultations. If you sense that your doctor is threatened by your intention to get a second opinion, then you might consider that to be further reason to pursue another perspective.

22. How do I go about getting a second opinion?

Unless you require emergency care, you should try to get a second opinion before starting treatment. Your doctor can advise you on how long you can afford to delay treatment. In the majority of cases, a few weeks won't make a difference to your health, and it makes sense to consider all options before making any treatment decision. There are also occasions after you have begun treatment when you may want to seek a second opinion; for example, if your disease is progressing and you are re-evaluating your treatment plan.

To guarantee an independent perspective, it is a good idea to seek a second opinion from a doctor associated with a different institution than your original doctor. Many insurance companies will pay for second opinions, but it may be worth paying out of pocket for a second opinion from a particularly well-qualified specialist, even if he or she is outside your plan. Arranging for a second opinion involves some logistics. You need to gather your medical records—including all reports and scans—to bring with you for a second opinion visit. You also will need to get your pathology slides. A second pathology opinion is typically part of the second-opinion process. If you are satisfied with your care but would just like to confirm your pathology, this can be done easily without an office visit. The Armed Forces Institute of Pathology is considered a leading pathology lab for second opinions. You can contact the AFIP by phone at 202–782–1630, or via their website at *www.afip.org.*

23. How can I relate best to my doctor? What can I do to make my medical visits as productive as possible?

The doctor–patient relationship lies at the heart of patient care. This relationship will guide and support you throughout the course of your lung cancer. It is your job, and your doctor's, to nurture this relationship and to work toward a partnership based on mutual trust and respect. Although difficulties between doctor and patient may occur at times, just as they do in any relationship, these problems will be minimized if good communication is maintained. Remember that your doctor is not a mind reader. It is your responsibility to be open and honest in your communications and to bring up any concerns, needs, or preferences you may have. It is especially important that you feel comfortable discussing sensitive issues such as your use of alternative medicine treatments, your lifestyle (smoking, drinking, drugs), end-of-life issues, and sexual concerns. Keep in mind that conversations between doctor and patient are confidential, and that the more your doctor knows about issues that may impact your health, the better care you will receive.

Your doctor is not a mind reader.

At your first visit you should address the issues of how much information you want from your doctor and how involved you would like to be in the decisions that are made about your care. Some patients want to know everything about their condition, and they want to make all the decisions themselves. Some patients find too much information anxiety-provoking. These patients would prefer to hear less information (often only the good news) and are more comfortable allowing their doctor to make all the decisions. Many patients fall somewhere in between. Whatever your preferences may be, and they may change over time, it is your responsibility to communicate them to your doctor. If you feel that your doctor is not responsive to your needs, or if you have other concerns regarding your relationship, you should bring them up before they reach a crisis stage. If you and your doctor cannot resolve disagreements in a productive and satisfactory manner, you should look for another doctor.

Think about what you are going to say to your doctor ahead of time. Remember, he or she has a finite amount of time to spend with you, so before your appointment consider which concerns are most pressing and write them down in order of importance. This tactic will help you focus and make the most effective use of the limited time you have with your doctor. Too often, patients spend time trying to remember if the nausea started on Monday, when Aunt Ellie was visiting for dinner, or on Tuesday, when they had Aunt Susie's casserole. If you choose to review events in great detail, you risk running out of the time that your doctor has for addressing your critical questions.

If you have symptoms to report, describe them clearly and concisely. Be prepared to answer your doctor's questions, such as when the symptoms started, how often they occur, and how long they last. Don't be afraid to mention the emotional and social issues that are affecting you, in addition to any physical problems you have.

Always bring someone with you to your appointment.

Always bring someone with you to your appointment. It is impossible to remember all that is said during an office visit, and emotions can cloud what a patient hears. It helps to have someone else along who can write down what the doctor says. Tape recording your conversations are another very helpful way of remembering exactly what transpired. As long as you tell the doctor what you are doing, most physicians have no problem with this. It is important that you understand everything that your doctor tells you. If something is unclear, say so, and ask questions until you are satisfied that you understand completely.

Be sure that all necessary tests are completed prior to your visit and that you have all the information you need. This includes having the required referrals, if any, and a current list of the prescription and nonprescription drugs you are taking. Bring a notebook or binder that contains your medical information and paperwork to each appointment. If you can present your doctor with the information she needs to care for you in an efficient and clear manner, you will go a long way toward increasing the quality of your relationship with your doctor and, ultimately, the quality of your care.

Emotional Aspects

24. How do I manage my emotions? Should I seek professional counseling? What types of psychosocial support are available to me?

A lung cancer diagnosis brings with it a tidal wave of emotions and a sense of uncertainty about the future. Feelings of shock, denial, anger, fear, helplessness, sadness, and anxiety are all normal responses to a life-threatening crisis. You likely will experience a range of emotions that will fluctuate from moment to moment and vary over the course of your disease. It is important to remember that there is no right or wrong way to feel and that it can take time to learn to cope with your emotions. You may hear from others that you can influence your chances for survival through positive thinking and an upbeat attitude. Although this approach may be helpful to you, you should not worry that feelings of anger or sadness will cause your tumor to grow faster—this is a common worry among cancer patients, but there is no evidence that it occurs. Expressing your emotions, both positive and negative, can be an effective way to relieve stress. You should feel comfortable using whatever coping mechanisms work for you and not be concerned about being a "perfect" cancer patient.

One method of coping that works well for many cancer patients is to reach out to others for emotional support. Spending time with family, friends, neighbors, and members of your religious community may help to reduce the sense of isolation brought on by your cancer diagnosis. In particular, connecting with other lung cancer survivors can be heartening and inspiring. People who are facing similar challenges share common concerns, experiences, and hopes for the future. The Alliance for Lung Cancer Advocacy, Support, and Education (ALCASE) provides a phone buddy program that will pair you with someone who has a similar type and stage of lung cancer. ALCASE also maintains a geographic listing of in-person lung cancer support groups. Support groups are not for everyone, but if you are looking for a community of people who will know exactly how you feel and can offer emotional support and practical information, a lung cancer support group will likely meet your needs. If no group is

There is no right or wrong way to feel; it can take time to learn to cope with your emotions.

Coping with Your Diagnosis

available in your area or if you are reticent to participate in an in-person group, you might consider joining
an online support group (also called a discussion list or
a mailing list). The Association for Cancer Online
Resources (ACOR) maintains four lung cancer lists: a
general list (LUNG-ONC), and specific lists for small
cell lung cancer (LUNG-SCLC), non-small cell lung
cancer (LUNG-NSCLC), and bronchioloalveolar carcinoma (LUNG-BAC). Online support groups are
especially valuable for patients who are physically
unable to attend in-person groups but who wish to
participate in a lung cancer community. (See Question
100 for information about locating lung cancer support groups.)

If you find that your distress persists and that you are
having ongoing difficulty managing your emotions, you
may want to seek mental health, social work, or pastoral
counseling. Your doctor can refer you to a psychiatrist
or psychologist who can evaluate your symptoms and
provide therapy to help relieve your distress. Clinical
social workers can also provide counseling and can alert
you to other sources of support. Mental health professionals can teach you coping strategies such as relaxation techniques and guided imagery. Your religion can
provide comfort at this time, and you may want to
approach your clergy about spiritual counseling.

25. How do I regain control of my life after my lung cancer diagnosis? How do I get past the emotional impact and move forward?

A lung cancer diagnosis can be overwhelming, making
it difficult to absorb information and focus on what
needs to be done. Your mind is clouded with thoughts

and worries about what your lung cancer will mean for you and your family. To move forward effectively, you need to make a mental adjustment. You need to redirect your energies toward the things you can control. Although you cannot change the fact that you have lung cancer, you can control how you respond to this challenge.

A first step toward gaining control of your thoughts is to realize that you are not alone in facing lung cancer. Thousands of people are surviving with lung cancer and leading happy, productive lives. The National Coalition for Cancer Survivorship defines a cancer survivor as anyone with a diagnosis of cancer. Cancer is not a death sentence. Many people view cancer as a chronic disease, something to be treated and managed. Keeping this concept in mind helps to make the cancer experience less frightening.

You are not alone in facing lung cancer.

Your new job is to become an involved cancer patient. The process of taking an active role in your heath care will help you to gain stability, confidence, and hope. Your efforts can make a difference in the quality of your care. Try to focus your energies on the following activities:

- **Adopting a healthy lifestyle.** Quitting smoking, maintaining adequate nutrition, and minimizing stress can all help your ability to fight your disease and withstand the effects of your cancer treatment (see Questions 84, 85, and 87).
- **Assembling a medical team.** You need to find doctors whom you can trust and who will provide you with excellent care. This may involve getting second opinions. You should keep in mind that good communication with all members of your medical team—

Coping with Your Diagnosis

including support personnel—is critical to the quality of care you receive (see Questions 20 and 23).

- **Gathering information and making informed decisions.** You need to learn all you can about lung cancer and its treatment so that you will understand what is happening to you. After gathering information and discussing your treatment options with your doctor, you will be able to make informed decisions about your care.
- **Learning to navigate the healthcare system.** Your doctor's office staff and hospital social workers can help you learn how to navigate the healthcare system. This will make your appointments more productive and minimize the aggravation over medical paperwork, insurance, and financial concerns (see Questions 29 and 30).

26. How do I cope with the stigma of having a "self-inflicted" disease? Should I feel guilty about my smoking? What if I never smoked—how do I cope with having a "smoker's disease?"

Your emotions following your lung cancer diagnosis are likely to be complicated by your feelings about smoking. If you were an active smoker, you may experience feelings of guilt. If you never smoked, or if you had stopped smoking years before, you may be shocked that you have been diagnosed with a smoking-related disease. This personal conflict over smoking is often exacerbated by the reactions of those around you and by the lack of public support for people with lung cancer. Some family members and friends may be angry with you for having caused your own disease. When acquaintances learn of your lung cancer, you may get tired of hearing the inevitable question, "Did you smoke?" And it is devastating to discover that the support services, media coverage, and fundraising events that are routine for other major cancers are rare for lung cancer. This lack of public empathy and support is demoralizing and adds additional stress to the challenges you face.

It is important to let go of any feelings of guilt. Guilt over smoking wastes energy that could go toward fighting your disease. Keep in mind that over 90% of smokers begin smoking as teenagers, at an age when the risks and addictive nature of nicotine cannot be fully comprehended. The tobacco companies continue to play an unconscionable role in perpetuating this deadly addiction among young people. In addition, they have specifically manufactured their cigarettes to be highly physically addictive.

One productive step you can take to help de-stigmatize this disease is to use whatever opportunities you have to put a face on lung cancer. Do not be afraid to speak up and identify yourself as a lung cancer survivor. The public needs to know that lung cancer affects everyone—mothers, fathers, sisters, brothers, and loved ones, young and old. It is easy to ignore lung cancer when "smokers" are cited as its victims. A "smoker" is an abstract notion, not a person with a life-threatening disease, worthy of caring and support. People with lung cancer have names, faces, and families, and they deserve the same respect afforded other cancer survivors.

You may get tired of hearing the inevitable question, "Did you smoke?"

People with lung cancer have names, faces, and families, and they deserve the same respect afforded other cancer survivors.

Coping with Your Diagnosis

27. What should I tell my children about my lung cancer? What if my children are grown?

Lung cancer does not just affect patients, it also affects their families and friends. Children are particularly vulnerable, and their welfare is often the primary concern of parents with lung cancer. Children should be told about a parent's illness. If things are hidden from them, or they are lied to, they will at some point sense that something is wrong. This may cause them to feel isolated or to fear that things are worse than they are. There is a good chance they will discover the truth anyway—either from overhearing conversations or from an unintentional slip—causing a loss of trust between parent and child at a time when that trust is so vital. It is better if they hear the news directly from a parent, so that it can be presented in a controlled and reassuring manner. In general, learning the truth about a parent's cancer will reduce a child's fear, even if the truth is frightening. It will remove uncertainty and enable the child to learn productive ways of coping with a difficult situation.

Before discussing your lung cancer with your child, you should give what you are going to say some thought, and try to anticipate questions your child may ask. Consider the following:

You do not need to tell your child every detail, but you should not lie.

- Children need information presented in a clear, understandable manner. Appropriate information will depend on the age and emotional maturity of the child. You know your child best. In general, you do not need to tell your child every detail, but you should not lie. You can be honest about uncertainty, but try to present the information in a realistic, yet hopeful, light.

- Prepare your child for what will happen next. If your child knows ahead of time that you will be having treatment and that you will experience side effects from your treatment (such as losing your hair or being very tired), he will be better able to adjust to your condition. It is helpful to stress that these effects are temporary.

- Reassure your child that someone will always be there to take care of him. Your child may worry about how your cancer will impact his life. It is important that your child's environment and activities be kept as normal as possible.

- Encourage your child to express his feelings and to ask questions. You may want to provide opportunities for your child to express his thoughts in writing or by drawing pictures.

- Let your child know that he may hear some frightening things about cancer, but that he should come to you to get the facts. You can tell him that while some people die from cancer, many people survive because they get effective treatments from their doctors. Stress that your doctors are taking good care of you and that you are getting the best treatments.

- Your child may want to meet your doctor. This can be a very positive experience. It can allow a child to feel more involved and to gain a more concrete understanding of what is being done to make you better. It is important that you take your cue about this from your child. No child should be forced to participate in anything beyond his comfort level.

- Let your child know that he did nothing to cause your cancer. If you smoked, you might anticipate a question about whether you caused your lung cancer by smoking.

It is a good idea to let your child's teachers (and the school psychologist, social worker, and/or guidance counselor) know about your lung cancer and family situation. These professionals can be extremely supportive during this time and can be alert to signs that your child may need extra help to cope with his feelings about your cancer. You should be aware that older children need as much support as younger children, and efforts should take into account the way your child expresses herself or himself in times of distress.

If you have adult children, what you choose to share with them about your lung cancer will depend upon the nature of your relationship. You will likely find that your children will react as you would have expected, but do not be surprised if your cancer causes them to act in ways you may not have anticipated. Even as an adult, it can be overwhelming to learn that one's parent has a life-threatening illness. If you find your children acting in ways that hurt you or make you uncomfortable (such as being overprotective or becoming emotionally distant), try to express your feelings and keep the lines of communication open. This becomes especially critical when your children do not live close to you, as is often the case with grown children. In particular, you will need to work out a system for relaying important medical information. You may feel comfortable handling this yourself, or you may have the person who accompanies you to doctor visits talk to your children about medical details. In any case, you should let your doctor know which family members you would like to be involved in your care.

Do not be surprised if your cancer causes your children to act in ways you may not have anticipated.

28. What do caregivers need to know to best support a person with lung cancer?

Caregivers play a vital role in the life of lung cancer patients, but they shoulder responsibilities that can be overwhelming at times. Demands placed on caregivers can be both emotionally and physically exhausting. To effectively support patients, caregivers must attend to their own needs, just as they attend to the needs of their patients. The following suggestions will help you to minimize the stress of the caregiving experience and become a more effective caregiver.

Educate yourself about lung cancer. Learn as much as you can about lung cancer, its treatments and side effects, and disease complications such as breathing distress. This will help you to understand what the patient is going through, and allow you to be a better cancer supporter and advocate.

Establish a relationship with the patient's doctor. The patient should let his doctor know that you are the primary caregiver. With the patient's permission, the doctor will answer any questions you may have. Be sure you understand your specific responsibilities for custodial care at home (such as dispensing medication, monitoring and reporting symptoms, and managing IV and oxygen therapy), and under what circumstances you should call the doctor's office for assistance.

Seek out help for daily tasks. Don't try to go it alone. Let family and friends know the work involved in being a caregiver, and identify specific ways that they might help you, such as running errands or spending

Coping with Your Diagnosis

time with the patient so you can take a break. If you can delegate responsibility for managing insurance paperwork to a trusted and competent person, this will relieve you of a significant source of aggravation.

Monitor your stress and health. Be mindful of how you are feeling, and try to address issues before you become overwhelmed. Set limits for what you can do and be sure to take time away from the patient to attend to your own needs. Remember: caring for yourself is as important as caring for your loved one. If you are not healthy, the patient will suffer, too.

Caring for yourself is as important as caring for your loved one.

Keep communication open. Providing emotional support is a critical aspect of caregiving. Often it is enough just to listen. You can and should talk about your own feelings and fears about the future. If you have anger over the patient's previous or current smoking, this is not a productive time to vent. The patient needs your unconditional support. It can be useful to discuss the changes in your relationship that have come about as a result of the patient's lung cancer diagnosis.

Seek out emotional support. Find people you can talk to about your experiences. This can be good friends or other family members. It is particularly helpful to find other caregivers who share your perspective and experience. You can often find support groups for caregivers and family members at hospitals, and through organizations like Cancer Care and the Wellness Community. The Association of Cancer Online Resources (ACOR) has an online support group for caregivers of people with cancer. (For further information on these resources, see the "support services" section of Question 100.) If you have persistent difficulties coping with your situation, you should seek professional counseling.

Focus on the positive. Although the challenges of caregiving are often daunting, the rewards are immeasurable. Caregiving is the greatest gift that one can give to a cancer patient. You gain the satisfaction of knowing that you actively helped your loved one in a time of need. Amidst the tedium, the aggravation, and the anguish are moments of tenderness and love that would not exist outside the cancer experience. If your loved one has limited time, you gain peace of mind that you have done the best you could to help him through his most difficult journey.

Caregiving is the greatest gift that one can give to a cancer patient.

Practical Aspects

29. What insurance and financial concerns do I need to address following a lung cancer diagnosis?

As difficult as it is to think about, newly diagnosed cancer patients must pay immediate and careful attention to insurance and financial concerns. The costs associated with cancer care can present an enormous economic burden. For the uninsured and underinsured, this financial strain can be devastating. Even for those who are well insured, cancer-related medical expenses can cause financial hardship. Inadequate insurance and insufficient finances can have a negative impact on the amount and quality of your cancer care, and on the course of your disease. Being proactive about your financial needs can help to minimize the cost and aggravation associated with your cancer experience, and insure that you can afford quality health care.

Your first step should be to examine your current health insurance coverage. Familiarize yourself with your policy and learn the scope of your medical coverage: What are your benefits? What are your restrictions? Are there circumstances under which you need pre-certification for coverage? Look at the sections on how to file claims and how to appeal denied claims. Try to anticipate what your medical needs might be, including the possibility for long-term care or hospice. Do you have adequate coverage in your current policy? If you do not have insurance or are underinsured, there are still options available to you despite your cancer diagnosis.

There are costs associated with cancer beyond health care, such as additional transportation and childcare expenses.

After assessing your insurance coverage, you need to examine your financial resources. Will you be able to comfortably pay all out-of-pocket costs? There are costs associated with cancer beyond health care, such as additional transportation and childcare expenses. You must also be prepared for the possibility that you may not be able to work for an indefinite period of time. Depending on your situation, you may need to convert your life insurance policy, retirement account, or other personal property into liquid assets. Now is the time to explore all potential avenues for financial assistance. You should get sound advice, and give careful consideration, before making any financial decisions. A financial counselor is best able to advise you on your current and future financial health.

There is a wide range of resources that you can turn to for assistance with your insurance and financial needs. Some of these resources include your doctor's staff, your hospital's social worker or financial counselor, your employer's benefits manager, and non-profit organizations such as the American Cancer Society, United Way, Cancer Care, and the Patient Advocate Foundation. These individuals and organizations can help you to navigate the complex insurance and managed care systems, provide direct assistance with your paperwork or finances, or refer you to additional sources of support in your community. They can lead you to services and programs, both private and government sponsored, that you may be eligible for and that may be useful to you. Some of these may include:

- additional health insurance through private carriers or government entitlement programs such as Medicare and Medicaid
- disability benefits (private, employment, state, social security)
- legal protections for getting and retaining health insurance coverage, preventing gaps in coverage, and for when you have been discriminated against due to your lung cancer
- allowable medical deductions on your income taxes
- Family Medical Leave Act (FMLA)
- Veterans Benefits
- specialized assistance programs for patients in need who require transportation for cancer care or access to free medications.

For further information on these organizations, services, and government programs, see Question 100. For an outstanding book that provides comprehensive, in-depth information on this subject, see David S. Landry's *Be Prepared: The Complete Financial, Legal, and Practical Guide to Living with Cancer, HIV, and other Life-Challenging Conditions,* published by St. Martin's Press (1998).

30. How do I learn to manage the medical paperwork? What are medical records, and what should I know about them?

Lung cancer generates a seemingly endless stream of medical appointments and paperwork. Handling the administrative tasks associated with your cancer care takes up substantial amounts of time and adds further stress to your already difficult situation. By understanding and organizing your medical information and paperwork, you will be better equipped to manage the logistics of your cancer care. This competence will help save you valuable time, reduce your aggravation, and generally increase your satisfaction with your health care.

Health information generated about you by your healthcare providers and your medical facilities becomes part of your medical record. Chart notes kept by your doctor, lab tests, CT scan reports, pathology reports, consultation reports, and hospital discharge notes are all examples of medical records. Medical records are used by your providers to plan your care and to communicate with each other. They are also used by insurance companies and legal entities to document your health care. Accurate health information compiled in a timely manner is essential for quality health care. Because mistakes are not uncommon, you should obtain copies of your medical reports at the time they are generated. Copies of chart notes are usually required when applying for social security benefits. In most cases, healthcare providers and medical facili-

Accurate health information compiled in a timely manner is essential for quality health care.

ties will accommodate patient requests for copies of medical records, although they may charge a small fee. (State laws vary on patient access to medical records. You can contact your state's health department to determine your rights.) The confidentiality of your personal health information is protected by law. Your medical records will not be shared with third parties without your authorization.

An effective way to manage the medical information and records that you will acquire during the course of your care is to use a three-ring binder with multiple dividers. This method of organization can be tailored to your needs, and the binder can be brought with you to every medical appointment. Binder sections might include personal information, medical information (including staging and treatment details), names of healthcare providers, reports (imaging, consultation, lab), pre-testing instructions, and insurance and billing records.

In addition to paper records, you need to collect copies of your imaging films, such as x-rays and CT scans. This is best done at the time of the study. Be sure to tell the technician *prior to your scan* that you would like duplicate copies of the films to bring home with you. In most instances, this request is easily accommodated. In some cases, you may have a delay in getting films (from a couple of hours to a day), and you may have to pay a small fee. Keep the films in an inexpensive portfolio, which you can purchase at any art supply store.

You may also need to access your pathology slides. These slides contain tissue specimens from your biopsy or surgery. You will need these slides when you are obtaining a second opinion. You can arrange with the hospital tissue bank or your doctor's office to obtain these yourself, or to have them sent directly to the consulting physician. It is helpful to know that the tissue bank also has your tumor block, which is an amount of your residual tissue that is generally kept for a number of years (this varies by institution), because there may be occasions when you need additional tissue specimens for further testing.

Treatment

What types of treatments are available
for lung cancer?

What is the difference between curative and
palliative treatment? How do I know what
the goal of my treatment is?

More ...

31. What types of treatments are available for lung cancer?

The three traditional treatments for lung cancer include **surgery**, **radiation therapy**, and **chemotherapy**. Lung surgery commonly involves an operation to remove the tumor, along with nearby lymph nodes (see Question 34). Radiation therapy (or radiotherapy) is the delivery of a beam of radiation aimed at the tumor with the goal of killing some or all of the cancer cells, thus shrinking the tumor (see Question 44). Both surgery and radiotherapy are local forms of treatment, which means that they only kill or remove the targeted tumor. Chemotherapy is a word for medications that kill cancer cells or stop their growth (see Question 39). Most chemotherapies are given intravenously (injected or dripped into the veins), but some are given orally. In either case, they get into the bloodstream and circulate around the body. Because blood flows through all parts of the body, in theory cancer cells anywhere in our body would be exposed to the chemotherapy. Therefore, chemotherapy is a systemic therapy.

There are always new treatments for lung cancer being tested in research studies known as clinical trials. You should familiarize yourself with the advantages and disadvantages of participation in clinical trials and explore the treatment options available to you through clinical trials (see Questions 57 and 58). If you are considering alternative therapies, such as herbal therapies, you should have an understanding of how to evaluate them. Alternative therapies are treatments not endorsed by the traditional medical establishment, because their effectiveness and safety have not been proven in rigorous scientific studies (see Question 61).

Surgery

Removal of tissue by means of an operation (surgical procedure)

Radiation therapy

treatment that uses high-dose x-rays or other high energy rays to kill cancer cells

Chemotherapy

the use of medicine to treat any disease, but especially for cancer

Intravenous

in the vein

32. What is the difference between curative and palliative treatment? How do I know what the goal of my treatment is?

Curative treatment is just what it sounds like—treatment given with the intent to cure the patient of his or her cancer. Typically, curative treatment for non-small cell lung cancer will include surgery, if the disease was discovered at an early stage. For Stage III disease (see Question 54), curative treatment may consist of chemotherapy and surgery, or chemotherapy and radiation therapy. For a limited stage small cell lung cancer, curative treatment usually consists of a combination of both chemotherapy and radiation therapy to the tumor in the chest. Treatment of advanced, metastatic non-small cell lung cancer is usually not curative, but **palliative**, in nature.

Palliative treatment is treatment that is given not with the intent to cure, but with the intent to prolong survival, shrink the tumor if at all possible, and improve the symptoms from the tumor. Realistically, chemotherapy for advanced non-small cell lung cancer is not curative. However, it is administered with the intent to shrink the tumor or at least keep it stable. In doing so, one hopes to prolong life and decrease symptoms, thereby improving quality of life.

Radiation therapy is an example of a treatment that can be either curative or palliative. Sometimes, in patients with local disease who are not candidates for surgery, high doses of radiation therapy can be administered with curative intent. More commonly, however, somewhat lower doses of radiation therapy are administered to shrink the tumor and reduce symptoms. Pal-

Treatment

Palliative treatment

treatment given not with the intent to cure but with the intent to prolong survival and reduce symptoms from the tumor liative radiotherapy is frequently given for brain metastasis, spinal cord metastasis, bone metastasis, and to the primary tumor in the chest. In these cases, it is usually effective at reducing the neurological signs and symptoms from the brain metastasis; alleviating pain from the bone metastasis and preventing further bone fractures; and ameliorating tumor-related symptoms, such as shortness of breath, cough, or bleeding.

It is appropriate to ask your doctor about the goals of treatment if he or she has not already told you.

33. What is performance status, and why is it important?

Performance status

the general condition of the patient

Performance status is a term used to describe the general condition of the patient. The general sense of wellbeing of the patient is an important prognostic factor; that is, patients who are relatively asymptomatic at the time of diagnosis, or who have mild or limited symptoms, are more likely to do well than patients who present very fatigued, weak, anorexic, and losing weight. There are several different grading systems for performance status; these include the ECOG (Eastern Cooperative Oncology Group) grading system and the Zubrich grading system. The ECOG grading system is rated on a scale of 0 to 4 and is defined in Table 2. The Zubrich grading system is defined on a scale of 100% to 0%, where 100% is totally asymptomatic and 0% is very near death.

Performance status is often used in defining eligibility for a clinical trial (see Question 57). Because patients with poor performance status are often very weak, most clinical trials exclude patients with a performance

Table 2   ECOG PS Grading System

PS GRADE	DESCRIPTION
0	Totally asymptomatic
1	Mildly symptomatic, able to perform daily activities
2	Able to perform daily activities with assistance, spends less than 50% of the day in bed
3	Needs considerable assistance for performing daily activities, spends greater than 50% of the day in bed
4	Totally bed-ridden, unable to care for oneself

Treatment

status of 2 through 4. There is, however, beginning to be more interest in defining appropriate, non-toxic treatment for these patients, and some clinical trials are being developed for performance status 2 patients.

Surgery

34. What is surgery for lung cancer? How is it performed?

Ideally, surgery for lung cancer should be done by a **thoracic surgeon** (see Question 19). The type of surgery performed is often dependent upon the stage of tumor, and the medical condition of the patient. The most typical operation is a **lobectomy** and mediastinal **lymph node dissection**. A lobectomy consists of surgical removal of the lobe of the lung that the tumor is located in. A mediastinal lymph node dissection consists of removing some or all of the mediastinal lymph nodes (the lymph nodes between the lung and heart). This dissection is often done to determine whether the

Thoracic surgeon
a surgeon specializing in chest surgery

Lobectomy
surgical removal of a lobe of the lung

Lymph node dissection
surgical removal of lymph nodes

tumor has spread to these lymph nodes. Occasionally, a patient may not be able to tolerate a lobectomy because underlying emphysema makes it too difficult for the remaining lung to keep the person alive. In these cases, a surgeon will sometimes do a **wedge resection**. This consists of removing the tumor itself and a small amount of lung tissue surrounding the tumor. A wedge resection will preserve more normal lung, but the chances of the cancer coming back are somewhat higher.

Occasionally, the tumor is located in an area such that all the lobes of the lung on that side are involved, meaning that they all contain some tumor. Sometimes the tumor is located in the largest airway on that side (the right or left main stem bronchus, which is the first major division of the trachea, the air pipe that delivers air to the lungs). If one of the main stem bronchi is involved, or if the tumor involves all the lobes on one side, a **pneumonectomy** must be performed. In a pneumonectomy, the whole lung is removed. Obviously, this is a much bigger procedure than a lobectomy or a wedge resection. Although a person with two normal lungs should be able to tolerate removal of one of the lungs without a significant impact on his or her breathing, very often patients who have been smoking and have a substantial amount of emphysema or bronchitis are not able to tolerate a pneumonectomy.

Typically, lung surgery involves an operation called a **thoracotomy**, which requires the surgeon to make a large incision to gain access to the lungs. Less invasive surgical techniques, such as video-assisted thoracoscopic surgery, are evolving and hold promise for

Wedge resection

surgical removal of the tumor and a small amount of lung tissue surrounding the tumor

Pneumonectomy

surgical removal of the entire lung

Thoracotomy

a common type of lung surgery that requires a large incision to provide access to the lungs reduced post-operative pain and complications and shorter hospital stays.

35. What determines whether I am able to have surgery?

To determine whether a patient is a candidate for surgery, three things must be established first:

1. Has the cancer metastasized? If the cancer has spread to other organs (Stage IV), a surgical cure is not possible and it does not make sense to do a large operation, considering the potential negative effects of surgery. Therefore, patients with metastatic disease usually do not undergo a curative resection.

2. The tumor must be resectable—that is, located in a place that the surgeon will be able to get to and completely remove. For example, if the tumor involves the heart, the surgeon obviously cannot safely remove the heart, and the tumor would be considered unresectable. In general, a tumor is considered unresectable if it involves any other major structures in the center of the chest, such as the heart, the large blood vessels going in and out of the heart, or the windpipe leading from the mouth to the lungs (the trachea).

3. The third criteria for surgery is that a patient must be healthy enough to withstand it. In particular, this involves evaluating two organ systems—the heart and the lungs:

    a.   The heart. If you have a history of heart disease, such as congestive heart failure, angina, or heart attacks, your surgeon will want to make sure that it is safe to operate on you, and that the stress of the surgery will not result in another heart attack. He or she may ask you to see a cardiologist, or heart doctor. The cardiologist will take a history, examine you, and may order an EKG, echocardiogram, or stress test before giving a final recommendation.

b. The lungs. Many patients with lung cancer are smokers or former smokers, and have some degree of emphysema or bronchitis (also known as chronic obstructive pulmonary disease, or COPD). If your doctor suspects you may have COPD, he or she will order **pulmonary function tests (PFTs)**. PFTs are a series of breathing tests that can help determine how healthy your lungs are and whether your remaining lungs will be able to support you if a portion of one of them has been removed. Your doctor may also order a preoperative quantitative perfusion scan, which is a nuclear medicine scan designed to predict how much lung function you will be left with after the operation.

Pulmonary function tests (PFTs)

a group of breathing tests used to determine lung health

36. What can I expect before surgery, and what can I do to prepare for it?

Prior to surgery, your surgeon will explain the procedure to you and arrange for an interview with either the anesthesiologist or a nurse anesthetist, who will go over your past medical history. You should be sure to disclose all of your medications at this time (including supplements, herbs, and over-the-counter drugs) so that the anesthesiologist can determine whether you need to stop taking them before surgery. Depending upon your health, the extent of the operation, and your hospital's policy, you may be admitted the night before the procedure. Many patients, however, come to the hospital the morning of the operation. You will be brought to the pre-op surgical suite, where you will change into a gown, and an intravenous catheter will be inserted into your arm. You may be given a medication to help you relax. (Keep in mind that this is something you can ask for if you are feeling overly anxious.) You will then be placed on a moveable cot (or gurney), and wheeled into the operating room. At first glance, this might appear to be a cold, sterile place where everyone is wearing surgical gowns, masks, and hats. The surgical staff, however, will likely make a concerted effort to see that you are comfortable. Once you are on the surgical table, the anesthesiologist will give you some medication into your vein to make you go to sleep. A tube will then be placed into your throat into which oxygen will be blown while you are asleep. You will sleep during the entire operation and wake up in the recovery room.

37. What does my surgeon mean when she says she "got it all"? Does this mean I am cured?

When your surgeon says she "got it all," what she is really saying is that she removed all the cancer she could see. The pathologist will look to see whether the biopsy sample or resected tumor from your surgery has **"positive margins."** Positive margins mean that the cancer cells extend to the very edge of the biopsy or surgical sample. If so, there is a high likelihood that there were tumor cells remaining on the other side of the sample—i.e., the side remaining in the patient. Even if your resected tumor has **"negative margins"** (normal tissue at the edge of the biopsy sample), there

When your surgeon says she "got it all," what she is really saying is that she removed all the cancer she could see.

Positive margins

a phrase used when cancer cells are found at the edge of the biopsy sample

Negative margins

a phrase used when normal tissue is found at the edge of the biopsy sample is no way to determine if there were microscopic amounts of cancer cells left behind either in the area of the tumor or somewhere else in the body. Unfortunately, none of the blood tests, x-rays, or scans currently available are able to detect microscopic amounts of disease.

Many patients whose cancer recurs after surgery are confused and angry because they remember their surgeons saying they "got it all." It is important to be aware that if your surgeon says she "got it all," she does not mean "there are no longer any cancer cells in your body, and you are cured." Although there is a considerable amount of research going on to detect smaller and smaller amounts of tumor, at this point the answer to the question "did the surgeon get it all?" is "we do not know."

Keep in mind that although successful lung surgery is reason to celebrate, you need to be vigilant about your follow-up care (see Question 90).

38. What should I expect following my surgery? What are the common complications of lung surgery?

When you wake up in the recovery room, you will be very "woozy" and might not realize where you are, or even that the operation is over. You will doze off and on while you are brought back to your room. For the first 24 to 48 hours, you may be uncomfortable, but the nurses should respond to your request for pain medications. You may also have access to **patient controlled analgesia (PCA)**, a method by which you can regulate your own pain medication. By pressing a but-

Patient controlled analgesia (PCA)

a method by which a patient can regulate the amount of pain medication he or she receives ton attached to an IV, you can give yourself a small dose of morphine. The PCA machine is set so that you will not be able to overdose yourself.

You most likely will have a chest tube when you come out of surgery. This is a tube leading from the space between your lung and chest wall to a bag or container by your bedside. Suction is applied to inflate the lung. In addition, you will probably have a catheter leading from your bladder to a bag by the bedside (a "Foley catheter"). This is painless, and will drain your bladder until you are able to go to the bathroom by yourself. Most likely, you will also have oxygen prongs or a face mask for supplemental oxygen.

Despite the IVs and catheters, the nurse will get you up out of bed the first day following your surgery. This is very important to prevent post-op complications, such as blood clots and lung problems. A lung that is not well ventilated is very susceptible to accumulation of secretions, which often leads to accumulation of bacteria and pneumonia. In addition, the nurse or respiratory therapist will give you lung exercises to do to prevent this complication. *It is important to have adequate pain control so that you feel like doing these exercises, so be sure to ask for and use pain medications as necessary* (see Question 74).

You will not be allowed to eat or drink until the doctors are sure your stomach and intestines have "woken up" following the surgery. Typically, a patient's GI tract tends to stop working for several days following a general anesthesia. When you start passing gas from below, you will be allowed to drink clear liquids. Your diet will advance as your stomach and small intestine become more active.

The most common complication following lung surgery is infection—usually a lung infection, often from
not breathing deeply and/or clearing secretions out of
the lungs. Other unlikely complications are bleeding,
infections of the incision site, and post-operative heart
problems, such as congestive heart failure or an irregular heart rhythm.

Make sure that you have adequate pain medications to
take home. It is not uncommon for surgeons to under-
estimate either the severity or duration of post-op
pain. Patients are often sent home with a small supply
of pain medication when, in reality, many will need to
take some medications for a month or longer. If your
doctor does not want to give you a large supply immediately, make sure you know how to contact him or her
for refills.

Chemotherapy

39. What is chemotherapy? How does it work?

Chemotherapy is medicine used to treat cancer. Unlike
surgery and radiation, which are used to treat localized
disease, chemotherapy is a systemic therapy used to
treat disease that has spread to all parts of the body.
Chemotherapy drugs are often administered intravenously (sometimes orally), and thus are absorbed
into the blood. Since the blood flows to all parts of the
body, in theory, cancer cells anywhere in the body
would be exposed to the chemotherapy.

Chemotherapy works by interfering with the DNA of
cancer cells (see Question 2). Because cancer cells

divide rapidly and exhibit uncontrolled growth, many chemotherapy drugs are specifically designed to target rapidly dividing cells. However, some normal cells in the body also grow rapidly—notably hair follicles, the lining of the stomach, and blood cells—and chemotherapy also affects these cells, causing unpleasant effects such as hair loss, nausea and vomiting, and immune suppression. In many cases, your oncologist will be able to provide you with supportive care to prevent or reduce these side effects.

Chemotherapy sometimes consists of one drug, but more often it involves a combination of drugs called a **regimen**. Chemotherapy regimens combine drugs that have different mechanisms of action, or ways of attacking cancer cells, in order to increase the effectiveness of the treatment and to prevent the cancer cells from developing resistance to chemotherapy. Your doctor will advise you on possible chemotherapy regimens based on your type of lung cancer, your stage, the location of your disease, your general health, your previous treatment, and the goals of your treatment plan. For information on specific chemotherapy drugs and regimens used to treat lung cancer, see p. 68.

Regimen

specific treatment plan; often used in reference to a combination of chemotherapy drugs (type of drug, dosage, and schedule)

40. What can I expect during chemotherapy?

The typical chemotherapy session begins with a standard blood test called a **complete blood count** (**CBC**). Because chemotherapy may have adverse effects on your blood counts, your oncologist wants to be sure that you are able to receive chemotherapy safely, without risk of infection or excessive bleeding caused by

Complete blood count (CBC)

a blood test that details the quantities of white blood cells, red blood cells, and platelets

Treatment

Chemotherapy Drugs for Lung Cancer

Chemotherapy recommendations vary depending on whether you have NSCLC or SCLC.

NSCLC

For NSCLC, **first-line therapy** (i.e., initial treatment) will often consist of two drugs, one of which is usually a "platinum" (cisplatin or carboplatin). Common regimens include: paclitaxel (Taxol) and carboplatin; gemcitabine (Gemzar) and cisplatin or carboplatin; vinorelbine (Navelbine) and cisplatin; and docetaxel (Taxotere) and cisplatin. In general, these drugs have roughly the same success rate in shrinking the tumor and prolonging life. However, they do have different side effects, schedules of administration, and cost, so many oncologists will base their decision on which one to use based upon these factors.

Should lung cancer progress during or following initial treatment, oncologists will often recommend a second-line therapy. The second line regimen for NSCLC that is approved in the U.S. is docetaxel (Taxotere). Oncologists sometimes use gemcitabine (Gemzar) if the patient did not receive it previously.

SCLC

For SCLC, first line therapy is often etoposide (VP-16) and either cisplatin or carboplatin. Recently, irinotecan and cisplatin has shown promise in treatment of extensive stage SCLC. Second line therapy for SCLC may include the following additional regimens and drugs: cyclophosphamide, doxorubicin, vincristine; carboplatin, etoposide (VP-16) and ifosfamide; and topotecan.

How to Learn More About Chemotherapy Drugs

It is best to discuss your chemotherapy alternatives with your oncologist since new chemotherapy drugs and regimens are constantly evolving. Your oncologist will be able to advise you on the likely side effects. If you are interested in further information about chemotherapy drugs, you can consult the following resources:

CLINICAL RESEARCH

To learn more about the effectiveness of lung cancer chemotherapies, you can search the medical literature via PubMed at: **www.ncbi.nlm.nih.gov/entrez/query.fcgi?db=PubMed** Enter the term "lung cancer" (use quotes) and the drug name in the search box separated by the word "AND" in all capital letters – for example:

| "lung cancer" AND carboplatin | **Go** |

You can further refine your search by clicking on the LIMIT button, which allows you to limit your search in various ways, such as by date, language, and type of publication.

SIDE EFFECTS

Ask your oncologist about the potential side effects of your chemotherapy regimen. He or she will be able to tell you what to expect and what to do if you experience side effects. MEDLINEplus, the National Library of Medicine's consumer health website, is also an excellent source of detailed information on chemotherapies and other drugs. For each drug, MEDLINEplus lists the brand name(s); a description; things to know before using the drug, such as allergy or pregnancy considerations; and a list of common, less common, and rare side effects. To access MEDLINEplus drug database, go to **www.medlineplus.gov** and click on "drug information." The Consumers Guide to Cancer Drugs (published by the American Cancer Society, 2000) provides similar information on chemotherapy drug side effects.

low blood counts. (See Question 42 for a full explanation of how chemotherapy affects your blood.) You can ask your nurse or **phlebotomist** (a technician trained to draw blood) to use a small butterfly needle for your blood draw, which will minimize the discomfort caused when the needle is inserted into your vein.

Phlebotomist

a technician trained to draw blood

The process of delivering IV chemotherapy is called an infusion. The most common IV method uses a thin needle or catheter (tiny plastic tube) that is inserted into a vein in your arm or hand. These IV needle sticks cause a bit more discomfort than a needle stick for a blood test because they require a slightly larger needle—the pain is a little sharper, but just as fleeting. Some patients apply a numbing cream (Emla) prior to needle sticks to make the process virtually painless. You may want to ask your oncologist or oncology nurse if this might be an option for you.

Once inserted, the needle or catheter is taped down to prevent it from moving and causing any pain. The chemotherapy drug(s)—and any pre-medications—are then dispensed from bags suspended from a metal IV pole. These liquids flow from the bags through a flexible tube that feeds into the needle or catheter in your vein. An infusion pump is sometimes used to deliver a precise amount of medication over a set period of time.

You will receive your pre-medications (pre-meds) first. These will likely include fluids for hydration and **anti-emetics** to prevent nausea and vomiting. Your oncology nurse should clearly explain the pre-meds and chemotherapy drugs you are getting. When the drugs begin to flow, you may feel a slight coldness or strange sensation at the IV site; however, the infusion process

Anti-emetics

drugs that prevent nausea and vomiting

should be pain-free and uneventful. If you experience pain, burning, swelling, shortness of breath, or any other unusual reactions during your infusion, you should bring it to your nurse's attention immediately. Your nurse will check to see if the needle was inserted properly, or perhaps adjust the flow of the medication to a more comfortable rate. There are other measures that can be taken to alleviate discomfort or other problems you may experience, so you need to keep your nurse apprised of your status.

The length of your infusion will depend on the number and amount of chemotherapy drugs you are receiving. Chemo sessions can take one hour, several hours, or several days. Extended infusions may require a hospital stay. For the duration of your infusion, it often helps to watch TV, read a book, listen to music, talk to a friend—do whatever relaxes you and makes the time go more quickly. When your infusion is over, be sure your nurse has told you about any potential side effects, what to do if you experience them, and under what circumstances you should call your doctor's office. If your nurse advises you that you may experience nausea, don't leave the office without a prescription for medications to prevent nausea and be sure you know how to use them.

In some instances, chemotherapy can be administered outside an office or hospital setting. Oral chemotherapies—in pill, capsule, or liquid form—can be taken by patients at home. Portable infusion pumps allow some IV chemotherapies to be delivered as patients go about their usual activities. These developments facilitate the treatment process and eliminate the inconvenience and distress associated with treatment visits.

41. What is a CVC or central line? What is a port? How do I know if I need one?

Patients typically receive chemotherapy intravenously through a thin needle that is inserted into a vein in the arm or hand. There are devices available called **central venous catheters** (**CVCs**) that allow repeated access to larger veins without the pain or stress associated with IV needle sticks into the smaller, more delicate veins. A CVC is a thin plastic tube that is inserted through the chest into a large vein near the heart. CVCs require minor surgery for insertion, but can be left in place indefinitely. There are two basic types of CVCs: external CVCs and ports (subcutaneous CVCs).

External CVCs. You may hear other patients talk about Broviac, Groshong, or Hickman catheters. These are names of common external CVCs. External CVCs are exposed through the skin to allow convenient and pain-free venous access for drawing blood and for delivering chemotherapy. They can also be used for blood transfusions, imaging contrast, fluids, and nutrition. External CVCs require periodic care to maintain proper function and to reduce the chance of blockage or infection. The risk of a clot formation can be minimized with the use of coumadin, a blood thinning medication.

Ports. Another option for convenient venous access is a port—also known as a medi-port or port-a-cath (Figure 2). A port is a type of central venous catheter that is implanted wholly under the skin. Ports provide

Central venous catheter (CVC)

a thin tube that is surgically inserted to allow access to large veins

External CVC

a type of central venous catheter that is exposed through the skin

Port

a type of central venous catheter that is surgically implanted under the skin

Figure 2   Schematic drawing of an implantable port. Reprinted from Yarbro CH, Frogge MH, Goodman M, Groenwald SL: *Cancer Nursing: Principles and Practice,* Fifth Ed. Copyright © 2000, Jones and Bartlett Publishers, Inc.

access to major veins but are not exposed through the skin as are external devices. They require no care and carry less risk of infection than external CVCs. Although needle sticks must still be made through the skin, the discomfort is less than with an IV needle stick because a special needle is used, and the skin over the port toughens and becomes less sensitive over time. Numbing cream (Emla) can be applied to make this process completely pain-free. Unlike external CVCs, ports are minimally noticeable—they appear only as a small raised area under the skin. Ports require general anesthesia for insertion.

Patients who should consider getting a venous access device include:

- patients who experience difficulty with blood drawing or chemotherapy IVs;
- patients who will be receiving chemotherapy on a frequent basis; and
- patients who will be receiving chemotherapy drugs irritating to small veins.

If you think you might benefit from having a venous access device such as an external CVC or a port, you should discuss this possibility with your oncologist. Most patients find that these devices greatly increase their quality of life during chemotherapy.

42. Why does my doctor order blood tests during my chemotherapy treatment? What are blood counts, and what should I know about them?

Because chemotherapy attacks rapidly growing cells, it has an adverse affect on the formation of blood cells. Your blood contains white blood cells, red blood cells, and **platelets**, each of which performs a specific function required for good health. If your chemotherapy treatment causes your blood counts (the quantities of your blood cells) to drop below normal levels, this can put you at risk for unpleasant and dangerous side effects. In some cases, these effects can be prevented or controlled through the use of supportive therapies.

Platelet

a type of blood cell responsible for clotting

To monitor the extent of the blood or hematologic effects of your chemotherapy regimen, your oncologist will order a test called a complete blood count (CBC). A CBC details the quantities and characteristics of each type of blood cell. Blood tests usually are performed prior to chemo, at times of low counts, and when low counts are suspected. Low blood counts may cause your chemotherapy treatments to be postponed or modified until supportive treatments (and/or the passage of time) bring them back to safe levels.

You should be aware of the following conditions caused by the effect of chemotherapy on blood counts:

Neutropenia: a low white blood cell (WBC) count.
White blood cells fight infection in your body. **Neutrophils** are one type of white blood cell that attacks bacteria. If your neutrophil count (called absolute neutrophil count, or ANC) drops to low levels, you are at higher risk of infection, including serious, potentially life-threatening side effects such as pneumonia. Neutropenia can be a dangerous condition for a cancer patient: infections in neutrapenic patients tend to be more severe than in other individuals and may necessitate hospitalization for IV antibiotics. If your counts indicate that your neutrophils are significantly below normal (a period called the **nadir** that usually occurs 10–14 days following treatment), you should avoid circumstances that might increase your risk of infection. Precautions you can take include frequent hand washing, avoidance of crowds (shopping malls, movie theaters, classrooms) or exposure to individuals with illness, and elimination of uncooked and undercooked foods from your diet. Neutropenia can be treated with drugs called **colony-stimulating factors** (such as Neupogen, Neulasta, and Leukine) that cause your bone marrow to increase production of white blood cells. If you experience fever, chills, sweats, or other symptoms of infection during chemotherapy treatment, you should contact your oncologist's office promptly.

Although neutropenia is experienced with all types of chemotherapy, the chemotherapy commonly used in lung cancer does not usually result in neutropenia that is so severe, or of such a long duration, that patients will come down with an infection. Fortunately, infection is relatively rare for lung cancer patients compared to other cancer patients.

Neutropenia
low white blood cell count

Neutrophil
a type of white blood cell that attacks bacteria

Nadir
lowest measured value; period of low blood counts

Colony-stimulating factors
substances that stimulate bone marrow to increase production of blood cells; also referred to as growth factors

Treatment

Anemia

low red blood cell count; may cause tiredness, weakness, and shortness of breath

Anemia: a low red blood cell (RBC) count. Your red blood cells carry oxygen to your body. A low RBC count means that there is not enough oxygen in your blood—you are anemic. Your oncologist may refer to a low hematocrit (the measure of RBC in your blood) or a low hemoglobin (a protein that is the primary component of RBC), two specific measures for anemia. If you become anemic, you may experience symptoms of fatigue, weakness, and dizziness; headache and shortness of breath can also be symptoms of anemia. Anemia may sometimes respond to treatment with erythropoetin alpha (EPO, Procrit). In some cases, a blood transfusion may be necessary to restore your RBC to safe levels.

Thrombocytopenia

low counts of platelets that may result in bruising and/or bleeding

Thrombocytopenia: low platelet levels. Platelets help to stop bleeding as they aid in clot formation. Patients with low levels of platelets may experience bruising or bleeding (e.g., nosebleeds, bleeding gums, intestinal bleeding). If necessary, transfusion of platelets can also be performed to restore platelet counts to normal levels. Although there is a drug called thrombopoetin that may help prevent thrombocytopenia, it has so many side effects that it is rarely used for lung cancer patients.

The effect of chemotherapy on blood counts varies widely among patients depending on the chemotherapy regimen and on the patient's individual response. Some patients experience only mild drops in blood counts and have few related symptoms. If you are aware of the possible effects (and associated symptoms) of chemotherapy on your blood, you will be able to identify potential problems, alert your doctor in a timely manner, and receive more effective treatment.

43. What are the common side effects of chemotherapy?

Although there are unpleasant side effects associated with chemotherapy, the reality is that most patients do not have terrible chemotherapy experiences. Invariably, tales of nausea and vomiting—among the most feared effects of chemotherapy—date from years ago when chemotherapy drugs were more toxic and when effective supportive care was not available. Advances in medicine have led to the development of chemotherapy drugs with fewer and less toxic side effects. Oncologists can now provide patients with supportive therapies such as anti-emetic drugs to prevent nausea and vomiting, medications to control pain, and growth factors to restore blood counts. It is important to remember that there is always something that can be done to eliminate, reduce, or help you cope with side effects from chemotherapy.

Advances in medicine have led to the development of chemotherapy drugs with fewer and less toxic side effects.

Another comforting thought is that almost all chemotherapy side effects are temporary and resolve immediately following treatment. It helps to remind yourself of this whenever you are experiencing distressing effects. Infrequently, there can be side effects that persist after treatment and never go away completely. Patients who experience severe **peripheral neuropathy**, for example, often complain that they have residual tingling and numbness in their fingers and toes years after chemotherapy. There are also a small number of adverse effects that may appear after treatment is completed—so-called "late effects." Although rare, these can be serious (second cancers are considered "late effects") and should be discussed with your oncologist prior to treatment. (See Question 83 for additional information on long-term and late effects.)

Peripheral neuropathy

tingling, numbness, or burning sensation in hands, feet, or legs caused by damage to peripheral nerves by a tumor or by chemotherapy or radiation

The particular side effects you experience will depend on which chemotherapy drugs you receive and your individual response. You should ask your oncologist or oncology nurse for information on the common side effects associated with your chemotherapy regimen. You need to be aware of how to manage the common effects and under what circumstances you should call your oncologist. Some patients find it helpful to keep a journal during chemotherapy treatment to record the dates, times, and duration of symptoms, along with descriptive information. The more accurate you can be in reporting your symptoms to your oncologist, the better care you will receive.

Although there are numerous side effects associated with chemotherapy, it is important to remember that no one gets all of them. In fact, most patients experience few side effects. Fatigue is the most pervasive side effect of chemotherapy. Other common chemotherapy side effects include:

- Hair loss (alopecia)
- Nausea and vomiting
- Drop in blood counts (white blood cells, red blood cells or platelets)
- Peripheral neuropathy

Less common effects:

- Oral effects: sore mouth and gums, changes in taste
- Gastrointestinal effects: diarrhea and constipation
- Infection
- Skin and nail problems
- Shortness of breath
- Loss of appetite
- Sexual effects: desire, fertility, hormonal balance

For additional information on side effects, see Part 5, Coping with Symptoms, Side Effects, & Complications (Questions 71–83).

Radiation Therapy

44. What is radiation therapy?

Radiation therapy (also sometimes referred to as radiotherapy, x-ray therapy, irradiation, or cobalt) is the use of high-energy rays to stop cancer cells from growing or multiplying.

45. How does radiation work?

Radiation affects normal and abnormal cells in the area being treated. It causes damage to the DNA, often irreparable, causing cells to die. After cell death, the cellular remains must be removed by the body's scavengers. This dead cell removal may be quite slow and there may be a delay in the shrinkage of irradiated tumors, even though all the cells are dead.

Radiation treatment is carefully planned to deliver as much radiation as possible to tumor cells while doing as little damage as possible to normal surrounding cells. Application in small doses over a long period of time increases the injury to the tumor cells while providing intervals between treatments to allow injured normal tissues to recover, thus reducing the side effects of radiation.

46. What is a "dose" of radiation? How many treatments will I need?

The "dose" of radiation is measured in units called **rads** or **Gray (Gy)**. The typical dose of radiation is 6000 rads or 60 Gy. (This is also equivalent to 6000 centigray,

Rad
unit of radiation

Gray (Gy)
modern unit of radiation dosage (older unit is a rad)

Centigray
unit of radiation

because one Gy = 100 centigray.) Rather than administer all 60 Gy in one treatment, the radiation is divided up into many treatments. The total dose of radiation and the number of treatments you will need will depend on the size, location, and type of your cancer.

Radiation delivered with "curative" intent usually consists of a total of 60 Gy given 2 Gy at a time, in 30 treatments or **fractions**. Treatments are typically given daily although occasionally there are specific reasons to give treatment more frequently (twice a day) or less frequently (two to three times a week). The standard course of radiation is given five days a week, Monday through Friday, over six weeks. There is some data to suggest that in certain situations, giving the radiation therapy twice per day for a total of 12 days may be more effective than standard fractionation.

Fraction

single treatment of radiation; a radiation dose is divided into fractions

The amount of radiation given to reduce symptoms is usually less than what is given in an attempt to cure the patient. This is because smaller doses of radiation can shrink the tumor enough to reduce symptoms and is associated with fewer side effects than "high dose" radiation.

47. What equipment is used to deliver radiation?

A variety of specialized equipment is used in both planning and treatment with radiation therapy. An x-ray machine called a simulator is used during the planning phase. A computer may also be used. The simulator and computer help determine the best plan for the treatment fields (areas).

The treatment may be delivered with linear accelerators or cobalt accelerators. Modern advances in the linear accelerator have made it the most commonly used equipment. A linear accelerator or "linac" produces high-energy x-rays. Instead of x-rays, the cobalt machines emit gamma rays. X-rays and gamma rays are very similar. Why one machine is chosen over the other is based on some technical factors of the machines and not on any difference in the effectiveness of the radiation beams in destroying cancer cells. The radiation oncologist's decision about which radiation-producing equipment to use is based on many factors, such as the type of cancer and its particular location in the patient.

48. What can I expect during radiation therapy?

The first visit to the radiation therapy department lasts one to three hours and usually does not include any treatments. A radiation oncologist will review your records and examine you to decide whether radiation therapy is appropriate and which treatment plan is best. He or she will discuss treatment recommendations with you, including how many treatments are needed and what their effects are likely to be. *This is the time to ask questions.* Your next appointment will be for a treatment planning CT or a simulation.

The purpose of the simulation visit is to plan the technical aspects of your treatments. A therapist will take you to the simulator room where they will accurately plan your radiation treatments. Simulators are not treatment machines; they are specialized machines built to mimic x-ray treatment units, and to take moving or still x-ray pictures. During your simulation, x-rays may be taken. In some cases a computerized tomography (CT) simulator is used to further refine treatment planning.

A variety of methods are used to line up your treatment field correctly. A special mold may be made for you to lie in during your treatment. Tiny dots may be tattooed on your skin to mark the center and corners of your field. These look like tiny freckles and will not be visible to anyone except those who know where to look. Oil-based markers or ink may also be used to mark your skin. It is important that you do not wash the marks off until all the treatments are completed. These marks stay on best if they are not allowed to get wet for the first 24 hours; after that period of time, you can bathe or shower. The water can run over the marks, but you should not use soap or a washcloth on the marked area. When the marks fade, the therapist touches them up at the treatment unit. The markings will rub off on clothes, so it's recommended that you wear older clothing. Pretreating the garment with a stain remover or hair spray before washing will generally remove the stain.

This simulation planning session usually takes one to two hours. You might get a treatment on this day, depending on whether special blocks need to be made for your treatment and whether there is an opening in the treatment schedule.

Most patients are treated on an outpatient basis. If you live too far away from the radiation center to commute from home, you might consider staying with local friends or relatives, or in a nearby motel. The treatment schedule can generally be tailored to accommodate at least a part-time work schedule.

49. What is the actual procedure like?

Radiotherapy treatments are very similar to having x-rays. Just as you are not able to see, feel, or hear the rays in a chest x-ray, there is no pain or discomfort with the actual radiation treatment. If you are in pain for other reasons, the treatment process may be uncomfortable because you will be required to lie still for a short period of time. Patients experiencing pain are encouraged to take pain medications one hour before a radiotherapy visit.

It is absolutely essential to remain in exactly the same position during the treatment so the radiation beam is always reaching the exact treatment area, rather than any surrounding tissue. Therapists use molds and other devices to minimize movement and to duplicate the identical position for each treatment.

A therapist will position you under the appropriate machine and then leave the room for the few minutes the machine is on. Because therapists work with radiation every day, it is essential that they leave the room during treatments to avoid getting too much exposure to radiation. The therapist does, however, stay nearby to monitor via television and can communicate with you through a microphone in the treatment room.

50. How long does each treatment take?

Treatments usually take about ten minutes each day. The machine is only on for about one minute for each treatment field; most people have at least two fields.

Patients can also expect some waiting time before their actual treatment. The treatment time may be longer if: 1) patients are treated on two different machines or have many fields, and 2) patients have a large field or a complicated set-up.

51. Are there advances in radiation therapy that I should know about?

Yes. Advances in radiation technology are allowing more effective treatment of tumor while decreasing the incidence of side effects. **Three-dimensional radiation therapy (3D-CRT)** is a technology that enables higher doses of radiation to be delivered to the lung tumor more precisely. This precision is accomplished by using a CT scanner to give a more accurate measurement of the tumor and its location. Thus, effective doses of radiation can be administered to tumors with less damage to normal tissue. A new type of 3D-CRT technology called **intensity modulated radiation therapy (IMRT)** is currently under investigation. IMRT promises to further increase the effectiveness of radiation treatment by using radiation beams of varying strengths. Tumors are irregular in thickness and shape, and IMRT technology can control the intensity of radiation delivered to different parts of the tumor, thereby increasing tumor kill and decreasing radiation-induced side effects. **Stereotactic body radiotherapy** is another high-precision technology under investigation for treatment of lung tumors.

Your radiation oncologist can tell you whether any of these technologies might be appropriate treatment options for you.

Three-dimensional radiation therapy (3D-CRT)

a type of radiation therapy that enables higher doses of radiation to be delivered more precisely than standard radiation therapy

Intensity modulated radiation therapy (IMRT)

a type of three-dimensional radiation therapy (3D-CRT) that uses radiation beams of varying strengths

Stereotactic body radiotherapy

a highly precise radiation therapy technique; when used to treat brain metastases, it is called stereotactic radiosurgery

52. What are the common side effects of radiation therapy?

To get to the tumor, the beam of radiation has to pass through all the tissues in front of and behind the tumor, thus generating side effects in these normal tissues. It is because of these side effects that radiation cannot be administered to the entire body; instead, it must be limited to the areas of tumor.

Some side effects of radiation are due to damage to normal tissues, which often takes the form of irreversible scarring (**fibrosis**). The amount of radiation that any one area of the body can tolerate varies. Tissues that are extremely sensitive to the effects of radiation include organs within the abdomen as well as the brain and spinal cord.

Fibrosis
scarring of the lung

The side effects of radiation relate to the amount and nature of normal tissues that the beam of radiation must pass through, as well as to the total dose of radiation given. Therefore, the side effects will vary from patient to patient depending upon the treatment plan for each patient. In general, however, common side effects of "high dose" (60 Gy, or 6000 rads) radiation on various body tissues are as follows:

- **Skin.** Radiation side effects to the skin can include a sunburn-like rash. For lung cancer patients, this is rarely a major problem.
- **Normal lungs.** Radiation can cause irritation of the lungs (**pneumonitis**), which can result in shortness of breath and cough. In some patients, this can result in permanent scarring of the lungs (fibrosis). Although these side effects are mild and well tolerated in most

Pneumonitis
irritation of the lungs

Treatment

patients, in some patients with underlying poor lung function, the resultant loss of breath is so significant that the patient ends up on oxygen permanently. Sometimes, the radiotherapist will prescribe steroids if he or she thinks radiation pneumonitis or fibrosis is the cause of the breathing problem.

- **Esophagus.** The esophagus is the tube through which food travels from the mouth to the stomach. Because it passes through the very center of the chest, it often gets exposed to radiation and can become irritated. Irritation of the esophagus usually manifests itself as a sore throat and difficulty swallowing, particularly solid foods. This is a temporary side effect that usually occurs three to four weeks into the radiation treatment, and continues for about two weeks afterwards. Rarely, this irritation may cause scarring of the esophagus, which can result in problems with food getting "stuck." If this happens, the patient may need an upper endoscopy, in which a gastroenterologist looks down into the esophagus with an endoscope, and then uses a balloon at the end of the endoscope to squeeze open the scar tissue and dilate the esophagus.

  If the sore throat experienced during radiation therapy becomes too bad, many radiation therapists prescribe a liquid medication that has some lidocaine in it. Lidocaine can numb the throat, making it easier to eat. During this period of time, do not worry about eating a balanced meal, meat, or solids. It is more important to stay hydrated and consume as many calories as you can, usually in the form of high-protein or calorie shakes, puddings, creamed soups, and the like.

  Recent studies in NSCLC patients undergoing chemoradiation treatment found that the drug amifostine (Ethyol) may reduce treatment-related esophageal symptoms. Ask your doctor if a radio-protectant, such as amifostine, is available to you.

- **Heart.** It is rare to experience heart toxicities from radiation. The radiotherapist is usually able to direct the beam of radiation so that only small areas of the heart are exposed.
- **Spine.** The spinal cord is very sensitive to radiation. Indeed, this is often what limits the amount of radiation that can be delivered, because side effects from spinal radiation are usually irreversible. Irritation of the spinal cord can cause back pain and, rarely, numbness, tingling, and weakness of one of the legs, which, in extremely rare cases, can lead to paralysis.
- **Fatigue.** Most people undergoing radiation therapy experience fatigue. It is important to get enough rest during this period. The fatigue usually subsides one to two weeks after the treatment is finished.

Combined Modality Therapy

53. What is combined modality therapy for lung cancer? What are the advantages and disadvantages of this approach?

Combined modality therapy usually refers to administering two types of treatment: a local treatment (such as radiotherapy or surgery) and systemic chemotherapy. This is usually recommended when a patient has locally advanced (Stage III) disease, although it is being explored more and more in Stage I and II lung cancer. Combined modality therapy is recommended because such patients are often at high chance of recurrence—either locally (at the site of the original tumor) or distantly (somewhere else in the body). In the latter case, distant recurrence is not a failure of the surgeon—presumably, at least some cancer cells must have metastasized before the operation. In the former case, again, a local recurrence does not mean that the surgeon did not do his or her job—it means that microscopic amounts of cancer cells, too small for the surgeon to see, were left behind. Therefore, two types of treatment are needed: therapy aimed at the tumor itself (surgery or radiation) and therapy aimed at cancer cells that might have already escaped (chemotherapy).

The subject of combined modality treatment, and how to administer it, is one of the biggest areas of controversy among lung oncologists. When should the doctor give the chemo? Before radiation or surgery? After? Which type of "local" treatment should you have—radiation or surgery? Both? Should the chemotherapy be given at the same time as the radiation? Which chemotherapy is best? Because medical knowledge regarding combination therapy is evolving, you should discuss the pros and cons of each of these approaches with your doctor (see also Question 67).

One of the potential disadvantages of combined modality therapy is enhanced side effects.

- Chemotherapy is probably better tolerated if it can be given before, rather than after, surgery. Patients are stronger and more likely to be able to tolerate the full chemotherapy treatment program that is prescribed.
- If high-dose radiation (60 Gy, or 6000 rads) is given before surgery, the normal tissues become so affected that the treatment area of the body has a hard time healing, and problems with wounds breaking apart inside the chest can result. Lower

doses of radiation (45 Gy, or 4500 rads) are better tolerated pre-operatively.

- Chemotherapy given concurrently with radiation instead of sequentially, in particular, is more difficult. Patients tend to experience many more problems with fatigue, sore throat, and swallowing. In addition, they are more likely to suffer from radiation pneumonitis and fibrosis (see Question 52). Nevertheless, because some oncologists feel strongly that there is a survival advantage when the treatment is given this way, it is often recommended, particularly for patients with good performance status.

Chemotherapy given concurrently with radiation instead of sequentially, in particular, is more difficult.

Treatment of NSCLC

54. What are the standard treatment options for my stage NSCLC?

The standard treatment of NSCLC depends upon several factors, including the stage of the disease and the patient's general strength. The first of these will influence which treatment will be recommended; the second will determine whether this treatment program needs to be modified.

Please note that the following treatment recommendations are generalizations only. You must talk to your oncologist about your specific case. He or she may modify these recommendations based upon the specific circumstances of your situation or your underlying health. In addition, advances in the treatment of lung cancer are being made everyday; what is recommended today (or in this book) may be outdated tomorrow. An excellent source for current information on lung cancer treatment is the NCI/PDQ Treatment Summaries, which can be found on the National Cancer Institute's web site, *www.cancer.gov*.

Stage I NSCLC

Stage I NSCLC is a tumor that is usually relatively small (less than 3 centimeters, or 1-1/2 inches) and does not involve any lymph nodes. The standard therapy for Stage I NSCLC is surgery, preferably a lobectomy if the patient's underlying function is adequate, and a wedge resection if it is not. With surgery, the chances of being cured of this cancer run between 60–80%. Some patients, however, cannot even tolerate a wedge resection because their lung function is so poor; other patients may have such significant heart disease that they cannot tolerate any operation. In these cases, high dose radiation can sometimes be given, although it is less likely to be curative compared to surgery.

Areas of Research/Clinical Trials (see also Questions 57–60)

Although most patients with Stage I lung cancer are cured of their disease, many are not. Lung cancer doctors are exploring two major areas of research for Stage I patients:

Chemopreventive agent

a natural or synthetic substance used to prevent cancer

Chemoprevention

the use of natural or synthetic substances to prevent cancer

• Can a **chemopreventive agent** prevent the development of lung cancer? In addition to their risk of recurrent disease, patients who develop one lung cancer are at higher risk of developing a second. This risk exists because the carcinogens in nicotine smoke are inhaled into both lungs and could have caused mutations in more than one place. **Chemoprevention** refers to the use of a substance, such as a drug or vitamin, to prevent the formation of cancer. There are several large clinical trials looking at the possible role of certain drugs as chemopreventive agents (see Question 96).

- Is **neoadjuvant** chemotherapy helpful? Neoadjuvant chemotherapy is a term for chemotherapy that is given before surgery to kill any microscopic metastases. It is given prior to surgery because patients are likely to be stronger and better able to tolerate it, and to attack the microscopic metastases while they are still small.

Neoadjuvant therapy

therapy given before the primary therapy; for example, neoadjuvant chemotherapy, which is sometimes given prior to surgery

Stage II NSCLC

Stage II NSCLC is a tumor that has spread to the local lymph nodes (also called hilar nodes, or N1 nodes) OR a tumor that is growing into the chest wall, but does not have any lymph node involvement. In both cases, surgery is the standard treatment of choice.

Areas of Research/Clinical Trials (see also Questions 57–60)

In addition to the research questions discussed above, another area of research interest for Stage II disease is the area of **adjuvant** therapy. Adjuvant therapy, in this context, refers to systemic therapy given following surgery for micrometastatic disease. Although "standard" chemotherapy has not been shown to be helpful, a number of new agents are being developed that may have more activity (see Question 60).

Adjuvant therapy

therapy given after initial treatment to increase its effectiveness; for example, adjuvant chemotherapy following surgery

Stage III NSCLC

Stage III NSCLC is a cancer that is big and bulky, and difficult or impossible to resect, but has no obvious signs of metastatic spread. It is typically subdivided into two sub-stages: **Stage IIIA,** which usually refers to a tumor that is technically operable from a surgeon's viewpoint, and **Stage IIIB,** which is not.

Stage IIIA

Common examples of Stage IIIA disease include:

- Mediastinal lymph node involvement (N2 disease)
- A tumor that is growing into the chest wall and has lymph node involvement (either hilar or mediastinal)

Stage IIIA disease is one disease stage for which combined modality therapy has definitely been shown to improve survival over single agent therapy alone. Again, clinical trials are ongoing to determine which of the following options is the best:

- Preoperative (neoadjuvant) chemotherapy followed by surgery
- Chemotherapy followed by radiation
- Chemotherapy given at the same time (concurrently) as radiation therapy
- Preoperative chemotherapy and radiation therapy followed by surgery

What has NOT been shown to be helpful is post operative chemotherapy (at least with "standard" drugs) and post-operative thoracic radiation. (Although post operative radiation therapy does not prolong survival, it probably helps prevent the tumor from coming back within the chest, and thus is commonly used for that reason.)

Stage IIIB

Common examples of Stage IIIB disease are:

- A tumor that is growing into the heart, trachea, or one of the large vessels leading into or out of the heart.

- A tumor with mediastinal lymph nodes on the other side
- Patients with a pleural effusion

In all of these cases, the surgeon cannot completely resect the entire tumor. If all of the tumor cannot be resected, surgery is generally NOT recommended. Surgery can be painful, is associated with some risk of complications, and is rarely curative in this situation. Therefore, it is generally thought that it is not helpful to operate on a patient's tumor unless you can "get it all." In addition, incision lines that contain residual tumor cells have a very hard time healing, so these patients are at increased risk for post operative complications.

Treatment of Stage IIIB disease usually involves chemotherapy and radiation therapy, except in the case of those patients who have a pleural effusion from the cancer. In these patients, the cancer cells probably involve the inside of the entire chest wall, which is too large an area to radiate (see Question 76). Therefore, patients with Stage IIIB disease with a pleural effusion generally receive chemotherapy alone, similar to patients with Stage IV disease (see p. 94).

Areas of Research/Clinical Trials (see also Questions 57–60)

The treatment of Stage IIIB disease is a very active area of research. Questions that are being explored include:

- Should the chemotherapy and radiation be given at the same time (concurrent chemoradiotherapy) or with the chemotherapy followed by radiation (sequential chemoradiotherapy)?

- If the chemo is given at the same time as the radiation, should it be given in standard doses (i.e., high doses every three weeks) or weekly, at lower doses? Should both high dose chemotherapy and weekly low dose chemo with radiotherapy be given, and if so, in what order? What are the best chemotherapy drugs for this situation?
- For those patients who have completed their chemoradiotherapy, and in whom the tumor appears to have stopped growing, is there anything else that can be given afterwards to prevent it from growing?

Stage IV NSCLC

Roughly half of all lung cancer patients will be diagnosed with either Stage IV (metastatic disease) or Stage IIIB with pleural effusion. Unfortunately, at this time, the prospects for cure from Stage IIIB or IV lung cancer are extremely remote. Therefore, the goals of treatment are to prevent the cancer from growing for as long as possible and reduce symptoms and, in doing so, improve both quality of life and survival. Because the cancer has spread, a local therapy is usually not recommended, unless it is to reduce specific symptoms (such as radiotherapy given to palliate a painful bony metastasis).

There are a number of different chemotherapy regimens used for the treatment of advanced NSCLC. They differ in terms of their side effects, cost, and how frequently they are given, but probably do not differ much in how well they work on the tumor. You should have a frank discussion with your medical oncologist regarding the pros and cons of the different regimens.

Treatment of SCLC

55. What are the standard treatment options for my stage SCLC?

Limited Stage

Limited Stage SCLC is potentially a curable disease. The optimal treatment consists of chemotherapy (usually four cycles) plus concurrent radiation therapy to the chest. However, as discussed in Question 53, this combination has significant side effects and probably should not be given to patients who are frail or who have bad lungs. Some physicians try to minimize the toxicity by giving the chemotherapy and radiation therapy sequentially instead of concurrently. In Limited Stage SCLC, this is probably not as helpful as giving them at the same time. At least one study showed that if the radiation therapy is given twice per day for 12–15 days instead of once per day for 20–25 fractions, patients are more likely to be cured.

Areas of Research/Clinical Trials (see also Questions 57–60)

Active areas of investigation include:

- What is the best dose of radiation therapy, and how should it be delivered?
- What is the best chemotherapy?
- Are there any other treatments that can be administered after the chemotherapy is done to prevent the cancer from coming back?

Extensive Stage SCLC

Although patients with advanced, metastatic SCLC are rarely cured, they very often respond to chemotherapy, at least for a while. The typical chemotherapy regimens in the past have been a platin (carboplatin or cisplatin) plus etoposide (VP–16). Recently there has been some evidence that cisplatin and a drug called irinotecan (CPT–11, Camptosar) may be better, but this data is somewhat preliminary and needs to be confirmed.

Areas of Research/Clinical Trials (see also Questions 57–60)

An active area of clinical investigation is identification of better chemotherapy regimens.

56. I have SCLC and my doctor has recommended prophylactic cranial irradiation (PCI). What is PCI, and how do I decide whether it is right for me?

Prophylactic cranial irradiation (PCI)

radiation to the brain with the intention of preventing the development of brain metastases

Prophylactic cranial irradiation (PCI) is radiation to the brain with the intention of preventing the development of brain metastases. It is based on the premise that chemotherapy does not penetrate well into the brain, so there may be micrometastases in the brain that have not been exposed to chemotherapy. PCI is recommended for SCLC patients who achieve complete remission following initial treatment because the brain is a common site of recurrence for SCLC. PCI reduces the incidence of brain metastases and improves both disease-free and overall survival for SCLC patients in complete remission.

The potential for mental impairment remains a primary concern for patients considering PCI. For most patients, this concern is unfounded. Although further research is needed, two large studies have shown that the long-term consequences of PCI on mental functioning are negligible.[1] The primary side effect of PCI is reversible hair loss.

If you are a candidate for PCI, you should discuss its pros and cons with both your oncologist and your radiation oncologist. An important question to ask is whether there is anything about you as an individual that puts you at risk for cognitive side effects. Although the risks from PCI are limited, certain patients may be more vulnerable to side effects. Another question to ask is whether PCI prevents you from having additional radiation therapy down the road should you need it. Because SCLC patients face a high prospect of brain metastases—which are associated with disabling symptoms and early death—the decision to undergo PCI makes sense in most cases when considering both quality of life and survival.

An important question to ask is whether there is anything about you as an individual that puts you at risk for cognitive side effects.

Investigative/Experimental Therapies

57. What are clinical trials?

Clinical trials are research studies involving people. Through clinical trials, scientists obtain knowledge

[1]Yang, G.Y., Matthews, R.H. (2000). Prophylactic Cranial Irradiation in Small-Cell Lung Cancer. *The Oncologist* 5:293–298.

The Yang article provides an excellent review of the literature on PCI. See also the opinion piece in the same issue:

Turrisi, A.T. III (2000). Prophylactic Cranial Irradiation in Small-Cell Lung Cancer: Is It Still Controversial or Is It a No-Brainer? *The Oncologist* 5: 299–301.

that spurs progress in fighting disease and improving health. There are many types of clinical trials (prevention, screening, treatment, quality-of-life) and an infinite number of questions that scientists can address by means of a clinical trial. The clinical trials process is designed to encourage rigorous investigation while protecting the volunteers who participate in the trials.

The clinical trials process for a new cancer drug begins with an application by the study sponsor to the Food and Drug Administration (FDA), the government agency that approves new treatments for marketing and sale to the public. The FDA provides oversight and approval for new drugs, new devices, new types of treatments, and new uses for established drugs, devices, and treatments. For most cancer trials, the study sponsor is either the National Cancer Institute (or one of its associated trial groups, including the Eastern Cooperative Oncology Group [ECOG], the Southwestern Cooperative Oncology Group [SWOG], the American College of Surgeons Oncology Group [ACOSOG], the Cancer and Leukemia Group B [CALGB]), or a drug company. The study sponsor must demonstrate that testing of the drug in laboratory studies ("in vitro" studies, meaning in a Petrie dish or flask) and in animal studies ("in vivo" studies) showed promise with a reasonable expectation of safety in humans. After the investigational new drug (IND) application is approved, an investigational drug will usually undergo three phases of testing, and ongoing FDA review, before it is eligible for final FDA approval:

- **Phase I trials** are designed to test the safety of the new drug. They are conducted in a small number of people (usually less than 50) who are given the drug in gradually increasing amounts to assess side effects and establish the most appropriate dose and schedule.

- **Phase II trials** determine how effective the drug is for treating a specific cancer in larger groups of people. Additional information on the nature and extent of side effects is gathered during Phase II trials. If the drug looks like it might have activity in a certain tumor type, then a Phase III trial is conducted.

- **Phase III trials** are designed to test whether a new drug is better than the standard treatment for a specific cancer. Both the effectiveness of the drug and the amount and extent of side effects are compared. The number of people participating in Phase III trials can range from hundreds to thousands.

Phase III trials frequently employ a trial design called a **randomized controlled trial (RCT).** In an RCT, the trial participants are randomly assigned (by chance, like the flip of a coin, although the randomization process is usually performed by a computer) to the treatment (experimental) group or the control group. You may hear these groups referred to as "arms." The experimental arm receives the new treatment alone, or the new treatment combined with standard treatment. The control arm receives the standard treatment. This process may be double-blinded, which means that both the patients and the doctors do not know who is in the experimental group and who is in the control group.

Randomization, control, and blinding are all scientific methods used to ensure that the trial results will not be biased in favor of one outcome or another. If clinical trials were not randomized, physicians might tend to

Randomized controlled trial (RCT)

a research study in which the participants are assigned by chance (using a computer or a table of random numbers) to separate groups that compare different treatments; a method used to prevent bias in research

Treatment

refer all of one type of patient or another to a particular arm of the study. For example, if the medical oncologist thinks a drug is particularly promising but is worried about side effects, given the option, he or she might decide to enter only the youngest patients to the investigational arm of the study, and enter the older patients to the control arm, thereby possibly biasing the results.

One type of trial design that concerns many potential trial participants is a placebo-controlled trial. A **placebo** is a dummy or inactive substance that is given to individuals in the control arm of certain trials. Some cancer patients avoid clinical trials for fear of getting a placebo. This fear is unfounded. It is extremely rare that a placebo-only arm is used in a cancer treatment trial. It is unethical to treat patients with a placebo when effective care is available, even if it is in the context of testing a promising new drug. The only circumstance in which a placebo-only arm is used in a treatment trial is if the standard of care for the type and stage of cancer being studied is no treatment at all. Your doctor will tell you if a study involves a placebo, but you should ask in any case.

Placebo

an inactive substance

58. How do I learn about clinical trials? How do I evaluate whether a trial is the right one for me?

Your first step should be to ask your oncologist whether a clinical trial might be appropriate for you. He or she may recommend a specific trial or trials and can discuss the pros and cons of your participation. You may also want to research clinical trials yourself to increase the chances that you have covered all of your options. (This task can be delegated to a family member or friend if you are not up to the effort.) Your oncologist will be able to help you evaluate what you find. (For information on how to locate clinical trials, see the clinical trials locators listed in Question 100.)

If your doctor does not have access to clinical trials, the next step is to contact the principal investigator, or study coordinator, of the trial itself. He or she will evaluate your eligibility for the trial by reviewing the inclusion criteria (for example, type and stage of lung cancer) and exclusion criteria (for example, some studies might exclude patients with kidney disease for safety reasons or require potential participants to have had no prior chemotherapy). Eligibility criteria are used to protect participants and also to ensure that the study participants are alike in certain ways so that trial results will be more reliable. After it has been determined that you are a potential candidate for the trial, the **informed consent** process begins. The process of informed consent is designed to protect your interests and safety as a trial participant in a scientific experiment by giving you the information you need to make an informed decision about whether to participate. The process begins when the investigator or study coordinator explains the trial to you. He or she will describe the purpose of the study, why you are eligible, how many people are participating, the procedures of the trial, the anticipated risks (which may include physical, financial, psychological, and legal risks in addition to any potential risks to your privacy/confidentiality), the costs of the trial, if any, as well as alternatives that may be open to you other than the trial. Your rights as a trial participant should be made clear:

Informed consent

a process that provides potential participants in a clinical trial the information they need to make an informed decision about whether or not to participate

Informed consent is designed to protect your interests and safety as a trial participant in a scientific experiment by giving you the information you need to make an informed decision.

that your participation in a clinical trial is voluntary, that there is no penalty for withdrawal, and that you are free to leave the study at any time. Before you sign the informed consent document, ask your doctor who will cover the costs of the trial, including the costs of treating any unexpected side effects. Be sure you understand everything and that you discuss it with whomever you trust to help you with your medical decisions.

An additional safeguard built into the clinical trials process is the requirement, prior to starting the any clinical trial, for review by the Institutional Review Board (IRB) at the institution where the study is conducted. The IRB is an independent committee of the hospital that makes sure that clinical studies meet ethical guidelines, and that prospective participants are given all the information they need to know in order to make an informed consent.

There are many good reasons why you might consider participating in a clinical trial: you may have exhausted the standard treatments available to treat your lung cancer; you may feel that standard therapies don't have much to offer you and that a new drug holds more promise; you may feel that you will get better care in a clinical trial; or you may want to help patients who come after you. Whatever your motive(s), you should be sure you understand the differences (in terms of risks, benefits, and practical considerations, such as time and cost) between a clinical trial and your other options. Only then can you make a truly informed decision.

59. What if I don't qualify for a clinical trial? Is it possible to get access to investigational (experimental) drugs and unapproved therapies outside of clinical trials?

Yes, it is sometimes possible to gain access to experimental drugs and unapproved therapies outside of clinical trials. Non-research access to investigational drugs is often called compassionate use, or special exception, and is determined on a case-by-case basis by the trial sponsor, subject to approval by the FDA. Compassionate use decisions are based on individual patient situations, drug availability, and other concerns. For NCI-sponsored trials, your doctor can make an application on your behalf to the Cancer Therapy Evaluation Program (CTEP). CTEP coordinates all aspects of clinical trials for the NCI, serves as a liaison to the FDA, and administers the NCI's non-research (compassionate) program. The general guidelines applied by CTEP in evaluating compassionate use applications are: 1) patients must have exhausted standard therapies and be ineligible for a clinical trials protocol; 2) there must be evidence that the experimental drug is active for the patient's disease (usually this requires Phase II data); and 3) the patient's doctor must determine that the patient is likely to benefit from the drug. For further information, contact CTEP by phone at 301–496–5725 or visit the CTEP web site at *www.ctep.cancer.gov/requisition/compassion.html*. For trials that do not involve the National Cancer Institute, or one of its affiliated trial groups, your doctor should contact the drug company sponsor directly.

It is sometimes possible to gain access to experimental drugs and unapproved therapies outside of clinical trials.

Expanded access programs are another way that patients can gain access to investigational drugs outside the clinical trials setting. Recently, an expanded access program was established by Astra-Zeneca for its investigational lung cancer drug Iressa (ZD1839) after the drug showed encouraging results and no major side effects in Phase I and Phase II trials. The expanded access program made Iressa available to patients who did not have access to, or qualify for, the Phase III clinical trials of Iressa, but whose disease had progressed or relapsed on standard chemotherapy. Expanded access programs for promising investigational drugs are available only infrequently and usually come about when a drug is awaiting final FDA approval for a serious disease or condition for which effective treatment options do not exist.

In cases of both compassionate use and expanded access programs, your doctor can advise you and will likely be your best advocate for obtaining non-research access to investigational drugs.

60. What are some investigative (experimental) treatments for lung cancer?

The past 10 to 15 years have seen an explosion in our understanding of "the biology of cancer"—what causes it, what makes cancer cells different from normal cells, what cancer cells need to live, etc. This explosion of knowledge has resulted in the development of new treatments based upon our increased understanding of the biology of the cancer. Many of these potential new treatments are just starting to undergo testing in clinical trials.

Unlike chemotherapy, which kills both normal (e.g., hair cells or blood cells) and cancer cells indiscriminately, many of these newer treatments are targeted at aspects of the cell that are specific for cancer—hence the term **targeted therapies.** A theoretical advantage of these targeted therapies is that they are specific for cancer cells and not normal ones; therefore, the side effects associated with them should be much less.

A number of different areas of investigation can be lumped under the term "targeted therapies." Some of these include:

- **Gene therapy**. As discussed in Question 2, genes are the thousands of subunits composing our DNA, which control the actions of our cells. Mutations in genes can cause the cells to behave abnormally. Scientists are discovering, somewhat surprisingly, that many different types of cancers have the same mutations in the same genes. Therefore, an active area of investigation aims to replace the abnormal genes in the cancer cells with normal ones **(gene therapy)**. This is done by directly injecting the tumor with the normal gene. Scientists are currently working on ways to inject the gene into the bloodstream so it can be taken up by cancer cells anywhere in the body.
- **Growth factor inhibitors**. As mentioned in Question 2, cancer cells are often stimulated to grow by substances called growth factors. One of particular interest is the epidermal growth factor (EGF). EGF is probably made by some cancer cells, and is secreted into the space surrounding the cancer cell and the rest of the cancer cells that make up the

Treatment

Targeted therapy
therapy directed at aspects of the cell that are specific for cancer

A theoretical advantage of these targeted therapies is that they are specific for cancer cells and not normal ones.

Gene therapy
treatment that replaces the abnormal gene in a cancer cell with a normal gene

Growth factor inhibitors
substances that inhibit the growth factors that stimulate cells to grow

tumor. In doing so, the EGF-secreting cancer cell stimulates its neighbors to grow. The EGF doesn't directly diffuse into a cell; instead, it binds to a receptor on the outside of the cell. Binding of the EGF to the EGF receptor (EGFr) activates the receptor, causing a chemical chain reaction that eventually ends up in the nucleus of the cell, stimulating the cell to grow. A number of different drugs are being developed to stop EGF from activating the receptor, and/or stopping the chain reaction that tells the DNA to start to grow and divide. Some of these drugs work by blocking the EGF from getting to the receptor (these are usually antibodies to the receptor and come in IV form); others work by preventing the activated receptor from sending chemical signals to the nucleus. Iressa and Tarceva are examples of this latter kind of drug, which usually comes in oral form. At this point, it is not known whether either approach is better than the other.

Angiogenesis
inhibitors

drugs that prevent
the formation of new
blood vessels

- **Angiogenesis inhibitors.** As discussed in Question 2, tumors need a constant and growing blood supply to feed them, much like an advancing army needs a constant and growing supply of food and materials to sustain it. Blocking off this blood supply should, in theory, have two effects: it should "choke off" the cancer by stopping the flow of oxygen and nutrients to it, and it should stop the tumor from spreading through its usual highway—the bloodstream.

COX-2 inhibitors

substances that
inhibit production of
proteins called
prostaglandins

- **COX–2 inhibitors.** COX–2 inhibitors, such as celecoxib (Celebrex), are related to the commonly used class of mild pain relievers, called nonsteroidal antiinflammatory drugs (NSAIDS), such as Motrin or Advil. Originally developed as pain relievers that would have lesser side effects on the stomach than NSAIDs, COX–2 inhibitors recently have been found in laboratory studies to slow or halt the growth of tumors in mice. This observed effect may occur because they inhibit the production of proteins called prostaglandins. Prostaglandins cause pain (which is why these drugs work as pain killers), and may also have a role in the formation of cancer. Numerous clinical studies evaluating these agents are underway, including the use of COX–2 inhibitors for chemoprevention of lung cancer (see Question 96).

In addition to targeted therapies, there are other new treatment methods under investigation for use in lung cancer:

- **Radiation.** Stereotactic body radiotherapy and three-dimensional conformal radiation therapy (3D-CRT), including Intensity Modulated Radiation Therapy (IMRT), are different methods of administering radiation that are more precise than traditional radiotherapy. Research is underway to determine the feasibility and effectiveness of these radiation techniques in the treatment of lung tumors (see Question 51).
- **Chemotherapy.** New methods of administering chemotherapy, such as inhaled chemotherapy and heated chemotherapy, are in clinical trials for treatment of lung cancer.
- **Photodynamic therapy (PDT).** PDT uses laser light to kill cancer cells that have absorbed photosensitizing drugs injected into a patient's bloodstream. PDT has been approved for treatment of both early- and late-stage lung cancer. It is used in advanced lung cancer to relieve symptoms caused when a tumor blocks an airway, such as shortness of

Photodynamic therapy (PDT)
treatment that uses laser light to kill cancer cells

breath and coughing. PDT is also effective for treating early-stage lung cancer in patients who are not candidates for traditional surgery. Trials are ongoing to determine additional uses for PDT in the treatment of lung cancer.

- **Radiofrequency ablation (RFA).** RFA uses high-frequency electric current to kill cancer cells. Clinical trials are underway to determine whether this method can be used effectively in the treatment of lung tumors and bone metastases.
- **Protectants/Sensitizers.** Active areas of investigation include research into drugs that can increase the effectiveness of lung cancer chemotherapy and radiation (sensitizers) or reduce treatment side effects (protectants).

These are just some examples of the many promising treatments being developed for lung cancer. For additional information about clinical trials and how to locate them, see Questions 57 and 58.

Alternative Therapies

61. What is alternative medicine?

Alternative medicine generally refers to therapies developed outside of mainstream medicine and used in place of standard, clinically proven therapies. Some of these therapies are touted as "cures" for cancer, with little or no scientific information to support them. It is often impossible to establish the reliability of individual testimonials, locate scientific research on alternative therapies, or verify the credentials of an alternative medicine practitioner. Unproved alternative therapies are often promulgated and sold by the same person, a charlatan who attempts to exploit vulnerable cancer patients.

Radiofrequency ablation (RFA)

treatment that uses high-frequency electric current to kill cancer cells

Insurance does not cover these types of alternative treatments. The cost of alternative medicine can be significant in terms of dollars, and in wasted time and energy. Most importantly, they can be dangerous to your health.

On the other hand, "alternative medicine" can also describe traditional medical systems, such as Traditional Chinese Medicine (TCM) or Ayurveda (from India). Although these systems have been in use for centuries, they have not been studied with the same scientific rigor as Western medicine. Because of this lack of data, many in the Western medical community view these alternative systems with skepticism and resistance.

When alternative methods are used in addition to conventional therapy, it is often referred to as complementary medicine. Although complementary medicine can include approaches such as herbal therapies, the term often refers to methods such as acupuncture and mind/body techniques (guided imagery, meditation) that are aimed at ameliorating side effects and symptoms rather than curing disease. Complementary methods can range from nutritional supplements and herbal therapies, to hypnotism and biofeedback, to art therapy and spiritual practices.

There has long been a disconnect between patients and doctors with regard to the use of complementary and alternative medicine (CAM). A significant percentage of patients use some type of complementary therapy but do not share this information with their doctors. Some patients feel that their doctors would not be receptive; others see no reason to tell their doctors.

A significant percentage of patients use some type of complementary therapy but do not share this information with their doctors.

Doctors often fail to ask patients about their use of complementary medicine. For some doctors this may reflect a bias against alternative methods or a lack of expertise; for others it may reflect an ignorance or lack of concern about the prevalence of CAM use among patients. Poor communication on CAM issues may compromise patient care. The good news is that there is more ongoing scientific research into CAM therapies, thereby encouraging awareness and dialogue on CAM issues. The National Institute of Health has established the National Center for Complementary and Alternative Medicine (NCCAM), dedicated to encouraging research and disseminating accurate information on CAM therapies. The National Cancer Institute's Office of Cancer Complementary and Alternative Medicine (OCCAM) supports the NCCAM mandate, focusing specifically on CAM for cancer.

62. What should I know about complementary and alternative therapies? How can I evaluate them?

You may be interested in learning about complementary and alternative medicine (CAM) treatments for a variety of reasons. Your current treatments for lung cancer may not be working and you may not see any effective treatments on the horizon. Maybe you are experiencing nasty side effects from standard treatments (like chemotherapy and radiation) and feel that CAM treatments such as acupuncture may provide relief. Perhaps CAM may represent philosophies that are more in line with your belief system than those of conventional medicine. Because the majority of CAM treatments have not been subject to rigorous scientific review, you need to be especially careful when considering

CAM therapies and providers. Here are some thoughts to consider:

- Talk to your doctor about CAM treatments. Even if your doctor is not receptive, he or she can advise you on potential side effects that you may not anticipate, such as the danger of massage for some lung cancer patients with metastases or low platelets. Your doctor can also alert you to circumstances in which your CAM treatments might interfere with your standard treatments, as in the case of megavitamins and chemotherapy/radiation. Because many doctors fail to ask their patients about CAM, it is important that you bring up this information yourself.
- If you are interested in pursuing alternative therapies, check the NCCAM (*www.nccam.nih.gov*) and OCCAM (*www3.cancer.gov/occam*) web sites first to see if there is evidence of safety and effectiveness. This should be done for both alternative and complementary treatments. You will find comprehensive fact sheets and summaries on individual therapies (e.g., antineoplastons, acupuncture, coenzyme Q10, dietary supplements) with links to both CAM clinical trials and CAM scientific literature. Another valuable resource for checking the reliability of alternative therapies marketed to cancer patients is Quackwatch (*www.quackwatch.com*). Quackwatch reviews the evidence and provides critiques of these therapies and should be consulted prior to undergoing any alternative treatment. Your doctor can help you to evaluate what you find in your research and advise you on whether a therapy or method might make sense for you.
- It is crucial to understand that herbal treatments and dietary supplements (vitamins) are not regulated by the Food and Drug Administration (FDA), and

Treatment

111

therefore any claims about anti-tumor efficacy have not been validated or reproduced by independent investigators. There are also reasons to be concerned about quality control, as well as issues of safety and effectiveness in these substances that you may consider safe. The best policy is to discuss the possible consequences of taking these substances with your doctor before you take them.

- Check the credentials of your CAM practitioner carefully. Ask for information on education, training, and membership in professional organizations.

Complementary therapies abound. Some patients find that activities such as meditation, guided imagery, yoga, and tai chi help them to relieve pain, stress, and anxiety, and increase their quality-of-life. There is little scientific data, however, that they are helpful in controlling cancer. For further information on the complementary therapies available to you, check with your hospital's patient center, or contact a cancer support organization such as Cancer Care or the Wellness Community.

Treatment of Special Populations and Conditions

63. I am 78 years old. Is there any effective treatment for me? Are there particular considerations for treatment of elderly lung cancer patients?

Age alone should not prevent you from receiving treatment for lung cancer.

Age alone should not prevent you from receiving treatment for lung cancer. Elderly patients can undergo chemotherapy, radiation, and/or surgery if their overall health allows them to withstand the stress of treatment. Your doctor will determine your ability to undergo treatment by assessing your level of function (called performance status—see Question 33) and any coexisting medical problems that may complicate or mitigate against some treatments. These circumstances are often a primary consideration when determining treatment options. However, it is important to recognize that your overall condition is a better predictor of your ability to tolerate treatment than your chronological age.

When a chemotherapy drug is given alone as treatment it is called monotherapy. Several chemotherapy drugs have been studied for use as monotherapies in elderly lung cancer patients with encouraging outcomes and fewer side effects than the standard multi-drug regimens. These chemotherapies include vinorelbine, docetaxel, gemcitabine, and paclitaxel. Although elderly patients with good performance status can undergo standard chemotherapy regimens involving multiple drugs, patients with less-than-optimal performance status are frequently ineligible for regimens involving multiple adverse effects. Single-drug regimens can be a good choice for these patients, offering less toxicity without sacrificing effectiveness. Some of the newer, experimental treatment agents may also be appropriate for patients with poor performance status because many of these agents target tumor cells and leave normal cells unaffected, resulting in fewer and less toxic side effects.

For lobectomy or wedge resections, age alone is not a risk factor, and functional elderly patients should not be denied these surgical options based on chronological age. When surgery involves removal of the entire lung (pneumonectomy), however, there is a considerable risk of post-op complications and death over the age of 70. Pneumonectomy in the elderly should be undertaken with great caution and consideration.[2] When feasible, video-assisted thoracoscopic surgery (VATS) offers a safer, less invasive alternative to traditional, open procedures for all lung cancer patients. For patients who are judged to be medically inoperable (due to poor performance status or coexisting illnesses), there are often alternative treatment options. For example, radiotherapy (with curative intent) has been used in elderly patients who are not surgical candidates, but who have early stage NSCLC that is potentially curable.

If you are elderly with lung cancer, you should be alert to any age bias on the part of your doctor—it is both inappropriate and substandard care to receive less aggressive treatment solely because of your age. Elderly patients who are in good health and have a good performance status face no greater risks from standard treatments based on their age alone. For those elderly patients with compromised performance status and/or limiting illness, there may be alternative treatment options available. Communication with your doctor is essential to learning all of your treatment options. Only then can you make an informed decision based on what is right for you—whatever your age.

64. Are there specific treatments available for bronchioloalveolar carcinoma (BAC)?

Bronchioloalveolar carcinoma (BAC) is a sub-type of adenocarcinoma, where the cancer tends to spread diffusely throughout the alveoli in the lung (see Question 3). This often gives a somewhat hazy appearance on a

[2]Dyszkiewicz, W., Pawlak K., Gasiorowski L. (2000). Early postpneumonectomy complications in the elderly. *Eur J Cardiothorac Surg* Mar; 17(3): 246–250.

chest x-ray, similar to a pneumonia, instead of a discrete tumor mass. The disease progression of BAC tends to vary somewhat from pure adenocarcinoma— BAC is considered slower growing and less likely to metastasize, although the overall prognosis remains similar to other types of NSCLC.

Currently, BAC is treated the same as adenocarcinoma and other forms of NSCLC. Because it is slower growing, chemotherapies may be less effective for BAC. As doctors learn more about the nature of BAC, more effective treatments are being investigated. There are clinical studies underway in the BAC patient population of gene therapy (p53), inhaled chemotherapy, and Iressa, a targeted therapy. If you have BAC, it makes sense to contact one of the principal investigators of the BAC studies. (See Question 100 for clinical trials locators.) Because BAC is relatively rare, most doctors do not have experience with BAC and cannot advise you on the particular concerns related to BAC. The principal investigators of these trials see more BAC patients than other doctors and may be a good resource for you, whether or not you decide to participate in a BAC trial.

65. My doctor told me that I have developed brain metastases. What are my treatment options?

There are several ways to treat brain metastases, and your doctor will advise you about which treatments may be appropriate in your individual case. Traditional surgery may occasionally be used to remove a brain metastasis, particularly if it is a solitary metastasis and the tumor elsewhere in your body is under relatively good control. More likely, you will be treated with radiation. Whole brain radiation may be used if you have numerous small metastases to shrink or eradicate the tumors. Stereotactic radiosurgery (pinpoint radiation) may be used alone or in conjunction with whole brain radiation when there are only a few small metastases. In some cases, chemotherapy and other treatments used to treat primary brain tumors have been used in patients with brain metastases, but there is no evidence that these treatments are effective in prolonging survival for lung cancer patients.

66. How are bone metastases treated?

If your lung cancer has metastasized to your bones, treatment will be aimed at reducing pain and strengthening the bone to reduce the risk of fractures. Common sites of bone metastasis are the vertebrae, ribs, hip, leg, and arm bones. Traditional radiation therapy to the involved area is effective for reducing pain. Occasionally, if the tumor has weakened the bone to where it is on the verge of breaking, surgery may be recommended to remove the bone tumor and stabilize the bone to prevent future breakage. Another method for treating bone metastases is drug therapy using a class of drugs called bisphosphonates. Aredia and Zometa are two different bisphosphonates used in lung cancer patients. Given intravenously, both Aredia and Zometa can alleviate pain, strengthen bone, and may also help to slow the progression of bone metastasis.

Evaluating Treatment Options and Outcomes

67. How do I decide on a treatment plan when I am faced with multiple options?

This is a difficult question. Talk with your doctor, and make sure you know all of your treatment options and that you understand the differences among them. Carefully weigh the pros and cons of each treatment, and evaluate your priorities. Many factors may influence your decision. These may include treatment survival rates, side effects and quality of life concerns, cost, time commitment, travel, and so on. If, for example, being home as much as possible is one of your top priorities, you would be less likely to choose a daily intravenous treatment than one that requires coming to the hospital only once every three weeks.

Your doctor will advise you on your options and make treatment recommendations based upon his or her medical experience and training, and on what he or she knows about you, your tumor, and your priorities. Many patients feel pressured and/or overwhelmed with having to make the decision and prefer to follow their doctor's recommendation. Other people like to be more actively involved in the decision-making process. Whatever your preference, the doctor–patient relationship is a critical component of the process. If you communicate effectively with your doctor regarding what you want from your treatment, it will allow him or her to provide you with optimal treatment advice.

68. How do I know if my treatment is working? What is the difference between partial response and complete response?

A partial response (or partial remission) is defined as an approximate 50% shrinkage of the tumor as determined by x-ray, CT scan, or physical exam. A complete response (or complete remission) is total disappearance of the tumor. Note, however, that neither a partial nor a complete response necessarily translates into "cure." It is common for a patient to have a temporary response, meaning that the tumor initially shrinks with chemotherapy but then starts to grow at some point. Presumably, the chemotherapy must have killed off the "sensitive" cancer cells, leaving behind a population of cancer cells that were more resistant to chemotherapy, and which eventually started to grow.

The "official" way to tell whether the treatment is working is to get another scan and see whether the tumor is shrinking. However, many patients can tell even before the scan is taken, because their symptoms from the cancer improve as the tumor shrinks.

69. What if my disease has remained stable during treatment?

If your disease is stable, it does not necessarily mean the treatment is not working.

If your disease is stable, it does not necessarily mean the treatment is not working. There have been many cases in which a patient's tumor never shrunk according to a CT scan, but never grew either. Presumably, in these situations the cancer cells must have been killed by the treatment but never disintegrated enough to make it look like the tumor was shrinking. Alternatively, the tumor on the scan could now contain a lot of scar tissue that formed from the treatment.

70. What happens if my disease recurs? How is recurrence treated? Is it possible to survive a recurrence of lung cancer?

Recurrence is something that every lung cancer patient fears. If you have experienced a recurrence, do not despair. Although cure following a recurrence is rare, long-term survival is not impossible. Try not to let yourself become overwhelmed or paralyzed by this news—it is almost always the case that you will have treatment options that can increase your survival. Discuss these options with your doctor, including clinical trials, of which there are many. Follow the same decision-making process as you did when you were initially diagnosed. Weigh the pros and cons of each option. Seek a second opinion if you are not satisfied with your care. Make informed decisions. When dealing with recurrent lung cancer, it is especially important that you communicate with your doctor regarding your changing needs and priorities.

Asking what to do if your tumor keeps growing during treatment is one of the hardest questions for patients with lung cancer. Obviously, talk to your doctor about what the alternative treatments are. If your prior treatment included surgery or radiation, is now the time to consider chemotherapy? If you have failed one chemotherapy regimen, there are now second line and even third line chemotherapy regimens available for lung cancer. Radiation can be used on a specific spot or tumor. Many patients decide to participate in clinical trials (see Questions 57 and 58) if their cancers do not respond to conventional treatment.

Asking what to do if your tumor keeps growing during treatment is one of the hardest questions for patients with lung cancer.

Consider your priorities once again, and ask yourself how aggressive you want to be. Each time the tumor grows after treatment, it tends to become slightly more resistant to chemotherapy. If aggressively attacking the tumor as much as possible is something you want to do, advocate for yourself. Ask your physician very specifically what the alternative treatments are. If he or she cannot provide any, seek a second opinion at an academic cancer center (see Questions 21 and 22).

Coping with Symptoms, Side Effects, & Complications

Why am I always exhausted?

More . . .

71. Why am I always exhausted? What can I do for fatigue? Will the fatigue go away after my treatment is over?

There are numerous possible reasons for fatigue, particularly while on chemotherapy. One that has become popularized in the lay literature recently is fatigue due to anemia from the chemotherapy. A blood test ordered by your doctor should indicate if your red blood cell (RBC) count is low enough to be the cause of the fatigue. If so, a blood transfusion, or weekly injections of the drug erythropoetin, should bring your RBC count up.

Another possible reason for fatigue is depression. Depression can manifest in many ways, not just an overwhelming feeling of sadness. Patients can feel despair, discouragement, lack of interest in activities they once enjoyed, change in sleeping patterns or eating patterns, and fatigue. Although anyone with cancer may experience some of these feelings some of the time, a person is clinically depressed when the depression is of such a magnitude that he or she is not able to enjoy any activities that normally bring pleasure. If you feel this might be a possibility, talk with your doctor. (See Question 72 for additional discussion of depression.)

A person is clinically depressed when the depression is of such a magnitude that he or she is not able to enjoy any activities that normally bring pleasure.

In many cases, however, there is no easily identifiable correctable cause of fatigue. Chemotherapy and radiation are tiring—be prepared for it. Manage it by getting the rest you need and by being proactive about reducing your activities. Consider cutting back at work to part time, if at all possible. Find out in advance what your company's policy is regarding medical leaves of absence. Pamper yourself—accept help from friends. Don't worry about a messy house. Explain to your family that your body is undergoing a change and that you will not be able to do as much for the next several months. If your family has a hard time accepting this, have them come to an appointment and discuss this with your doctor.

72. Could I be depressed?

Depression is a common condition in lung cancer patients. Although patients who have a history of depression are most susceptible, many people who have never before experienced psychiatric problems may develop depression following a lung cancer diagnosis. Even though it is normal and natural to feel sad and down about the diagnosis, sometimes the feelings of sadness become so overwhelming that they take on a life of their own and become a problem in and of themselves. Patients can become so discouraged, hopeless, or full of despair that they are unable to enjoy their family or the little things in life. If you find yourself sitting at home all the time, no longer interested in your usual activities or in getting out of the house, withdrawing from your family, spending all your time in bed, and so on, you may be depressed. The good news is that most depression is treatable—and with medications that are usually well tolerated with minimal side effects. The bad news is that it frequently goes undiagnosed. Several factors complicate the process of diagnosing depression in cancer patients. The first is that many of the symptoms of depression (such as changes in eating and sleeping habits) are also symptoms associated with cancer and its treatment. Second, medical factors (such as high levels of calcium in the blood) and some anticancer treatments can cause depression. And third, patients often do not openly share emotional symptoms—a major component of the depression diagnosis—with their doctors. If you think you might be depressed, it is very important that you discuss this possibility with your doctor. If your doctor does diagnose depression, she can treat you or refer you to a psychiatrist for further evaluation and treatment. Most frequently, cancer patients have reactive depression. Reactive depression is of limited duration and can be helped with counseling. Major depression is more severe and long lasting, and treatment most often includes medication, such as antidepressants. When depression is treated effectively, patients experience relief of distressing symptoms and are better able to cope with their cancer and the demands of cancer treatment. Early recognition of the signs of depression will facilitate prompt diagnosis and successful treatment.

Early recognition of the signs of depression will facilitate prompt diagnosis and successful treatment.

Sometimes patients are unwilling to undergo treatment for depression, thinking that it represents a sign of weakness, and that they should be able to control their feelings. Nothing could be further from the truth. When you are hungry, you cannot trick your mind into thinking you are not. When you have to go to the bathroom, you cannot trick your mind into thinking you do not. If you are depressed, why would you be able to trick your mind into thinking that you are not?

73. Can my shortness of breath be controlled?

Pericardial effusion

accumulation of fluid inside the sac (pericardium) that surrounds the heart

There are many causes of shortness of breath, and management will depend upon the cause. For example, if the shortness of breath is due to a pleural or **pericardial effusion**, the fluid can be removed to restore breathing capacity (see Question 76). Shortness of breath caused by emphysema or COPD can be managed with inhalers and antibiotics, and pneumonia with antibiotics.

There are several ways to relieve shortness of breath if it is due to the tumor obstructing an airway. Radiation is often used to reduce the tumor, thereby relieving the obstruction. If the patient has already had maximal radiation, a **stent** can sometimes be placed. A stent is a device that looks similar to a hollow tube, which is inserted via bronchoscopy into the airway that is being blocked or crushed by the tumor. Other ways of relieving the obstruction include **brachytherapy**. Brachytherapy is a method of delivering a "seed" of a radioactive agent into the tumor that is blocking the airway.

Sometimes shortness of breath cannot be controlled using these methods. In these cases, the patient's shortness of breath can be managed symptomatically with:

- Oxygen. Portable oxygen carriers are available that allow patients to be mobile.
- Medications, particularly morphine. Morphine reduces the uncomfortable sensation of breathlessness, so although a person's body is not getting enough oxygen, the brain does not interpret it this way. Morphine can be given in a number of ways (see Question 74).
- An anti-anxiety medication, such as lorazepam (Ativan), will also help to relieve your feelings of breathlessness.

74. What can I do to relieve my pain?

First and most importantly, talk to your doctor. He or she cannot know you are in pain unless you speak up. Advocate for yourself: if one medication is not effective in relieving your pain, or is having a lot of side

Stent

a hollow tube that can be inserted via bronchoscopy into the airway to prevent it from being blocked or crushed by the tumor

Brachytherapy

internal radiation therapy that involves placing "seeds" of radioactive material near or in the tumor

You deserve to have relief from pain.

effects, tell your doctor. Do not wait until your next appointment—give the office a call. If they do not call back within a reasonable period of time, call again. You deserve to have relief from pain, and your doctor and nurse would agree with you if you let them know.

Everyone feels pain differently. Your doctor and nurse will often ask you to rate the pain on a scale of 1 to 10, with 0 being no pain and 10 being very severe pain. Some patients agonize over this question, struggling with the difference between a four or a five, and they should not. There is no wrong or right answer, and your nurse or doctor will not quiz you regarding fine differences. This pain scale is simply a general way to determine whether your pain is getting better or worse.

There are many medications for pain. Typically, physicians manage mild pain with non-opioid medications, such as acetaminophen (Tylenol), or nonsteroidal anti-inflammatory drugs (NSAIDS), such as Motrin or Advil. Some type of opioid is usually required for moderate pain. Commonly used preparations include combinations of acetaminophen or NSAIDs with oxycodone or hydrocodone (e.g., Percoset and Roxicet), administered every six hours. Severe pain may require morphine or hydromorphine. Sometimes patients with severe pain may need to be hospitalized for intravenous morphine to quickly control the pain and to determine how much oral morphine they will need as an outpatient.

Unfortunately, misconceptions about pain medications can sometimes prevent patients from taking these drugs or even talking to their doctor about pain relief. Some common misconceptions include the following:

- **I'm afraid of getting addicted to morphine.**

Don't be. Numerous studies have shown that cancer patients in pain do not get addicted to these drugs. They do not exhibit drug-seeking behavior and are able to go off the medications without difficulty once the cause of the pain is controlled.

Cancer patients in pain do not get addicted.

- **I want to save morphine for when the time comes and I will really need it.**

Don't. Numerous studies have also shown that patients do not become "tolerant" to these drugs—that is, they do not find themselves requiring more and more pain medications for the same level of pain.

- **OK, but I'll still try to get away with taking as few pills as possible.**

Don't. These pain medications are much, much better at preventing pain than taking it away once it starts. These pain medications are designed to be taken on a regular basis, whether you are having pain at that time or not.

Pain medications are much, much better at preventing pain than taking it away once it starts.

- **Won't morphine make me woozy and lightheaded?**

It might, but these are side effects that usually go away with repeated treatments. If you have this problem, try starting at a lower dose and slowly working your way up to allow your body to get used to it. If this doesn't work, tell your doctor, and he or she will try a different preparation. Although very variable, some people have more of one kind of side effect on one type of pill but not another.

• **I'm afraid to take morphine because codeine makes me so constipated.**

This is one of the major problems with these drugs. It is extremely important to try to prevent the constipation—it is much harder to correct constipation after it has already occurred. Talk to your nurse or doctor about the various types of medications recommended to prevent constipation. Typically, most patients start by taking a laxative or stool softener at the same time that they take their pain medications. If you become constipated, try adding milk of magnesia. If that does not work, ask your doctor about taking the same type of medications that are used in preparation for a colonoscopy, such as sorbitol, "Go-Lytly," or magnesium citrate.

When using these medications, it is important to know that this is an area where the "art" of medicine comes in. Everyone is different, so "play around" with the timing, amount, and combinations of these medications until you have a combination that works for you.

• **What are other side effects of codeine and morphine?**

Another common side effect is nausea. Like the constipation, if it cannot be managed with medications, ask your doctor to switch you to another type of preparation. Itching is a relatively rare side effect that can also be usually managed with medication.

• **What is the difference between codeine and morphine?**

Codeine, morphine, oxycodone, hydrocodone, etc., all fit into a class of very similar drugs called opioids. The codeine derivatives—codeine, oxycodone, hydroco-done—tend to be less potent than morphine or its derivatives (hydromorphine, Dilaudid), which simply means that you have to take more of them to get the same effect. They all have the same side effects, though.

• **What is the maximum dose of morphine someone can take?**

The short answer is there is no one maximal dose—it depends on the individual. The side effect that eventually limits the amount of these medications one can take is **respiratory depression**—slowing of the breathing. However, most people are able to tolerate very high doses of opioids as long as the dose is increased gradually. A dose that would have very severe side effects in a person who has never taken these drugs may not faze a person who has been on them a while. So, even though patients do not become "immune" to the pain killing properties of these medications, with time, they often become tolerant of the side effects.

Respiratory depression
slowing of breathing

• **I hate taking pills, period.**

Ask your doctor about a "fentanyl patch." This is a small piece of a plastic-like tape that contains a medication called fentanyl (or Duragesic). This medication gets absorbed through the skin over a 72-hour period of time, so the patch needs to be changed about once every three days.

• **What is the difference between oxycodone and Oxy-Contin?**

Oxycodone is a short-acting preparation of codeine—its effects usually last about six hours. OxyContin is a brand name for a long-acting preparation of oxycodone. There are a number of long-acting pain preparations, including OxyContin, MS Contin, Oromorph, among others. All of these medications are coated with a special substance that allows the medication to be slowly absorbed over many hours. The advantage of these medications is that they can greatly reduce the number and frequency of short-acting pain pills one has to take.

For these medications to work well, they have to be taken on a regular schedule. Because they get slowly absorbed, it may take several days for them to start to work. In the meantime, you can continue to take your "short-acting" pain pills. Indeed, many people have to take a short-acting pain pill occasionally for "break-through" pain.

Because they take longer to work, you may not feel any effects from these medications for a day or two. Therefore, it is important to take these medications whether you are having pain or not. Like their short-acting counterparts, the long-acting preparations are better at preventing pain than at relieving it, and because they take so long to work, you do not want to suffer tomorrow for not having taken one today. One way of looking at this is that the pill you take today will not be felt until tomorrow.

- **I'm afraid to take these medications, especially Oxy-Contin, after all the stuff I've read about in the newspapers.**

Don't be. Opioids, when taken for the appropriate reasons by conscientious individuals, are not harmful or addicting and are true "miracle drugs" for relieving pain. They only become problematic or addicting when used inappropriately for their side effects.

OxyContin in particular has been in the press lately. OxyContin is oxycodone (the same medication found in Percoset or Roxicet), but it is somewhat more concentrated. It comes in a preparation that allows the drug to be released slowly over 8 to 12 hours. Some addicts are breaking the pills open and then taking the amount of opioid that is intended to be used over 12 hours all at once. When used appropriately, these drugs are very helpful for lung cancer patients.

75. Am I at risk for a blood clot? What is a pulmonary embolism?

A blood clot that occurs in a deep-lying vein in the leg or pelvis is known as a **deep vein thrombosis (DVT)**. If the blood clot breaks off and travels up through the heart and into the lungs, it is called a **pulmonary embolism (PE)**. A pulmonary embolism is a potentially serious condition, because if it is a large blood clot, it can block off a blood vessel going to the lung and cause significant problems with breathing, or even death.

Deep vein thrombosis (DVT)

a blood clot occurring in a deep-lying vein in the leg or pelvis

Pulmonary embolism (PE)

a blood clot that travels to the lungs causing full or partial blockage of one or both pulmonary arteries

Lots of things can cause DVT, particularly in the elderly, including poor circulation, sitting for long periods of time, or being bedridden following surgery. For unclear reasons, cancer patients have a higher tendency to get blood clots.

To prevent DVT from happening, your doctor may put you on an anticoagulant (anti-clotting drug), such as coumadin (Warfarin) or heparin. These drugs do not cause the blood clot to dissolve. Instead, they prevent

Symptoms, Side Effects, & Complications

the blood clot from becoming even bigger, allowing it to shrivel up and become "glued" to the wall of the vessel. Although coumadin can work well in some cancer patients, in others it does not. Those patients often need to be treated with heparin. Heparin can be administered in several ways. Until recently, patients were often admitted for intravenous heparin. More recently, low-molecular-weight heparin has become available, which can be administered once or twice per day subcutaneously. Please note that the commonly used phrase "thinning the blood" is not quite accurate. These medications make the blood less likely to clot, allowing the body to take care of the clot as described above.

76. What is a pleural effusion and how is it managed?

A pleural effusion is a collection of fluid between the outside of the lung and the chest wall (the **pleural space**). The lung is covered with a thin membrane called the **visceral pleura,** and the inside of the chest wall is covered with a thin membrane called the **parietal pleura.** Normally, the outside of the lung is up against the chest wall. However, if there are tumor cells on either the visceral pleura, or the parietal pleura, they can become "irritated" and cause fluid formation.

Other conditions besides cancer can cause fluid accumulation in the pleural space, including congestive heart failure or pneumonia. To prove that the pleural effusion is indeed due to cancer, your surgeon will sample some of the fluid so it can be examined under a microscope by the pathologist. This is typically done by numbing the

Pleural space

the area between the outside of the lung and the inside of the chest wall

Visceral pleura

a membrane surrounding the lung

Parietal pleura

a membrane lining the chest wall

skin with a topical anesthetic, and then inserting a small needle into the chest and draining out some of the fluid.

One of the reasons pleural effusion is significant for lung cancer patients (in addition to the breathing problem it can cause) is that it exists in a "free-flow-ing" space. For example, when you stand up, the fluid settles to the bottom of the lung. When you lay on your side, it follows to the side and "layers out" along the side. If you were to stand on your head, it would flow to the top of the lung. As it flows, it can spread any cancer cells that might be floating within it, thus "seeding" other areas of either the visceral or parietal pleura. Because the fluid spreads the cancer cells around so extensively, local therapy, such as surgery and radiation, is usually not possible.

In most people, accumulation of some fluid in this area is not a problem. Some people, however, can experi-ence shortness of breath, particularly if the pleural effusion is quite large. When it gets large, patients may also experience an uncomfortable sensation of fullness or discomfort in the chest, as well as a cough.

The pleural effusion can be removed in an outpatient procedure called a **thoracentesis** (Figure 3). In this pro-cedure, a needle is inserted in the back between two ribs. It is attached to a tube that drains the fluid into a bottle or bag. The procedure is relatively painless. The skin is numbed with lidocaine before the needle is inserted, so you will feel the needle to numb the area. After that, most patients do not feel anything, with the possible exception of a cough or vague discomfort if a lot of fluid is removed. These effects are due to the lung re-expanding.

Thoracentesis

a procedure that uses a needle to remove fluid from the space between the lung and the chest wall.

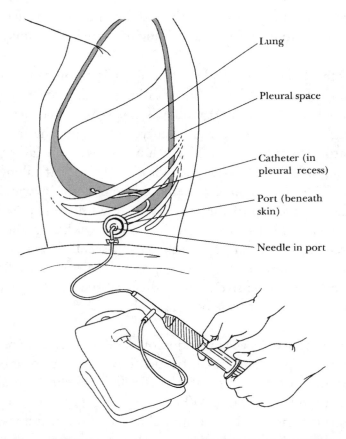

Lung

Pleural space

Catheter (in
pleural recess)

Port (beneath
skin)

Needle in port

Figure 3   Thoracentesis via an implanted port. Reprinted from Yarbro CH, Frogge MH, Goodman M, Groenwald SL: *Cancer Nursing: Principles and Practice,* **Fifth Ed. Copyright © 2000, Jones and Bartlett Publishers, Inc.**

Pleurodesis

a procedure to prevent recurrence of pleural effusion by draining the fluid and inserting medication into the pleural space

If the fluid keeps reaccumulating, your doctor may recommend a procedure called **pleurodesis**. Although there are several ways of doing this, they are all based upon the principle of draining the lung very, very dry, and then inserting some medication into the space where the fluid once was between the chest wall and lung. This medication is supposed to irritate the covering of the lung and the inside of the chest wall, which in turn is supposed to cause scar tissue (or fibrosis) to form between the two, thus serving as a type of "glue" to keep the surfaces stuck together. There are a number of different ways of doing this; the size of chest tube, the choice of medication, and whether the tube is inserted in the operating room or at the bedside will vary depending on local practices.

Regardless of exactly how the procedure is done, there are several points to keep in mind. First, the procedure doesn't always work. This may be because it is impossible to get the pleural space dry enough, or because sometimes the lung will not re-expand. In addition, it often involves between 5–10 days in the hospital, usually with a chest tube inserted, in order to get the pleural space as dry as possible. For these reasons, most oncologists do not recommend pleurodesis unless it becomes clear that a patient is going to need repeated thoracentesis.

77. I have heard stories from patients who underwent chemotherapy years ago and had terrible nausea and vomiting. Will I have a similar experience?

Almost certainly not. The good news is that a new class of anti-emetic drugs has been developed over the past decade that is much more effective in preventing nausea and vomiting. This class of anti-emetics, called HT3 blockers, can be given orally or intravenously. These drugs have had a major impact on the ability of doctors to administer—and patients to tolerate—chemotherapy. Even the "worst" chemotherapy drugs these days often only result in some queasiness and loss of appetite for a day or two. Vomiting is much more uncommon than it has been in the past. The bad news

Even the "worst" chemotherapy drugs these days often only result in some queasiness and loss of appetite.

is that these drugs are very expensive, particularly if taken orally, as some insurance companies do not pay for oral medications. Most oncologists will give these medications intravenously with chemotherapy, making chemotherapy considerably more tolerable than it was in the past. However, everyone is different. If you are unusually sensitive to the nausea side effects of chemotherapy and have problems with repeated vomiting episodes, call your doctor or nurse. Do not wait for your next visit! It is important not to become dehydrated—this will only make you feel worse, result in less fluid intake, and start a downhill spiral. If you call while you are having the problem, your doctor or nurse will alter your medications, and may even have you come to the office to receive anti-emetics intravenously.

78. Will I lose my hair during chemotherapy or radiation? What can I do to make the experience more tolerable?

Alopecia
hair loss

Hair loss, also known as **alopecia,** is one of the most common and dreaded of all cancer treatment side effects. Hair loss is difficult because it takes away your normal appearance and provides a constant reminder that you have cancer. You may feel that you are not yourself without your hair, and you may be uncomfortable or self-conscious around other people, even your family. It helps to remember that in the vast majority of cases, treatment-related hair loss is temporary, and there are things you can do to minimize the emotional and physical impact of losing your hair.

Hair loss occurs because both chemotherapy and radiation treatment adversely affect hair follicles, and other fast-growing normal cells, in addition to cancer cells.

With chemotherapy, your hair loss can range from a noticeable thinning, to patchy loss, to complete hair loss—or your hair may not be affected at all. The degree and nature of your hair loss will depend primarily on the type and amount of chemotherapy you are receiving. Your oncologist will be able to tell you what to expect, although to some extent the amount of hair loss varies from person to person. Ask your doctor which chemotherapy agents are more likely to cause hair loss, and which are not, and tell him or her if this is important to you. If you do lose your hair, it will begin to grow back about a month after your last treatment and take several more months to grow back fully. You shouldn't be surprised if the hair that grows back is a different texture or color than your normal hair. A change in texture is common, although over time your hair will most likely return to its original state. Extended chemotherapy treatments may also result in the loss of your body hair. This phenomenon presents additional challenges—for example, your nose will run frequently and sweat will drip in your eyes. For some people, the loss of eyebrows and eyelashes is more disturbing than the loss of hair, which is more easily camouflaged.

With radiation, you will experience hair loss only in the area that is irradiated. Your hair will usually grow back, although it may be thinner than it was previously. Your hair loss may be permanent if you receive high doses of radiation.

There are several things you can do to make your experience with treatment-related hair loss more tolerable. The first thing is to prepare ahead of time. You may want to cut your hair to a short style to make the transition less traumatic. If your hair loss begins with a gradual thinning, you can reduce the rate of loss by avoiding the use of heat (curling irons, hair dryers, hot rollers) or chemicals (bleach, dyes, perms, harsh shampoos), and by using a soft brush. If your hair begins to fall out in clumps, you may find it easier and less upsetting to just shave your head at that point.

If you are planning on wearing a wig, try to get one before you start chemotherapy so you will have it when you need it. Your oncology nurse or hospital social worker may be able to help you locate a wig shop that caters to the needs of cancer patients. Be sure to ask about the different types of wigs available and the advantages and disadvantages of each. It is possible to take your wig to your hairdresser and have it styled to look like your natural hair so that when you do make the transition, it will be less noticeable. Wigs vary greatly in cost depending on the quality of the wig you select, but your oncologist can give you a prescription for a "hair prosthesis" that will cover some or all of the expense if you have insurance coverage. A wig is considered a deductible medical expense. If you cannot afford a wig, the American Cancer Society, Cancer Care, and other cancer organizations provide wigs free of charge to those in need.

There is a wealth of choices for head coverings, including hats, scarves, and turbans. The American Cancer Society's Tender Loving Care catalog (800–850–9445 or *www.tlccatalog.org*) is a wonderful resource for these items and others designed specifically to hide hair loss. Keep in mind that there are no rules for what you should wear on your head, if anything, and you should do whatever is most comfortable for you.

Another excellent resource for learning to cope with hair loss, is the "Look Good...Feel Better" program (*www.lookgoodfeelbetter.org*) that is offered at the American Cancer Society and certain other nonprofit organizations. The program offers workshops in skin care, makeup, hair and nail care, and the use of wigs and headwear. They provide many useful tips for coping with head and body hair loss and provide free samples to take home. If you are not comfortable attending the program yourself, a friend or relative can go for you, or you can ask to see the program video.

Understanding that your hair loss is temporary and that there are things you can do to minimize the effects of hair loss will help you to get through this tough time.

79. I have numbness and pain in my fingers and toes that my doctor calls peripheral neuropathy. Is there an effective treatment for this condition?

Unfortunately, the short answer is no. Peripheral neuropathy occurs when peripheral nerves (the nerves located outside of the brain and spinal chord) are damaged. This condition can be caused by your tumor, but in most lung cancer patients it is usually caused by certain chemotherapy drugs, such as paclitaxel (Taxol) or cisplatin. Symptoms of peripheral neuropathy may include feelings of "pins and needles," numbness, and burning in the hands, feet, and legs. Motor disturbances such as dropping things or problems walking, can also result from peripheral neuropathy. Sometimes a drug called Neurontin can help, but this drug also has its side effects, such as fatigue. Some patients report that exercise helps with peripheral neuropathy and improves quality of life. In general, although the neuropathy rarely goes away completely, it can slowly improve with time. See Question 100 for resources to consult if you experience peripheral neuropathy.

80. Is my cough something I should worry about?

Cough is a common symptom that can be due to a number of causes, including lung cancer, infection, smoking, and asthma, among others. If you have a persistent cough, you should tell your doctor. Be prepared to tell him or her how long you have had your cough, when and how often your cough occurs, whether your cough produces mucous (and if it does, what color the mucous is), and whether your cough is associated with shortness of breath and wheezing. In the majority of cases, your doctor will be able to diagnose and treat your cough effectively with therapy specific for its cause. Persistent coughs can range from a minor annoyance to a major source of fatigue and discomfort for lung cancer patients. Because there is effective treatment available for most coughs, and because cough may be a symptom of a serious condition, it makes sense to seek medical attention for persistent cough. If at any time you cough up blood or see blood in your sputum (i.e., the mucous and other material that you cough up from your lungs), you should call your doctor's office immediately.

If you have a persistent cough, you should tell your doctor.

81. Will treatment for lung cancer make me infertile? Will it affect my sex life?

Chemotherapy can cause temporary or permanent infertility. If you think you may want to have children in the future, it is extremely important that you discuss this issue with your doctor prior to treatment. Factors that may affect fertility include the type of drug(s), the amount of drug you receive, the duration, and your individual response. Your doctor can advise you on your likelihood of infertility and on any steps that you might take to preserve your ability to have children—such as freezing your eggs or sperm for future use. Your doctor can also tell you whether you have any treatment alternatives that will not threaten your ability to have children. Radiation and surgery for lung cancer usually do not affect fertility, although to the extent that they reduce lung function, they may affect a woman's ability to carry a child. Some of the treatment agents currently in clinical trials for lung cancer do not affect fertility; however, the fertility effects of some experimental agents may be unknown. There may be nothing you can do to preserve your ability to have children in the face of lung cancer. If you share your concerns about this vital issue with your doctor, then he or she will be better able to advise you on your choices and help you to make these difficult decisions.

Your lung cancer impacts all aspects of your life, including your sexuality. A lung cancer diagnosis may affect how you feel about yourself sexually and how your partner feels about you. The pain, fatigue, shortness of breath, and other effects of cancer and its treatment affect you physically and emotionally and most likely will have a negative impact on your sex life. Communication is your best ally for combating this undesirable side effect. Communicate with your partner to let him or her know how you are feeling and how your disease and its treatment are affecting you sexually. Ask questions of your partner to be sure that he or she is expressing his or her feelings about changes that may be occurring as a result of your cancer. Discuss what you can do to accommodate these

Your lung cancer impacts all aspects of your life, including your sexuality.

changes, such as making mental adjustments or devising alternatives to compensate for physical limitations. Talk to your doctor to learn whether there are things you can do to ameliorate the symptoms that are interfering with your usual sex life. If your sexual relationship with your partner becomes a source of stress or concern, do not hesitate to discuss this with your doctor. Emotions and fear about cancer can cause you or your partner to make wrong assumptions or act in ways that result in hurt feelings. They can contribute to poor communication or exacerbate problems that existed prior to your lung cancer diagnosis. If you and your partner are having difficulties dealing with how your cancer is affecting your sex life, do not hesitate to seek professional counseling.

82. What can I do if I have lost my appetite?

Loss of appetite is a problem for many cancer patients. Some things to consider:

- Eat small meals more frequently (rather than three meals per day).
- Although it is always best to eat a well-balanced meal, for cancer patients who are struggling with loss of appetite, consuming calories is probably more important. Concentrate on eating high-calorie and high-protein foods. There are a variety of nutritional supplements available; many patients feel that they taste better cold, and may mix them with ice cream or pudding.
- Talk to a nutritionist.
- There is a medication called Megace (megesterol) that can help stimulate the appetite. Ask your doctor about it.

83. Are there long-term effects from treatment?

Your cancer treatments cause side effects. Many of these effects are temporary and disappear shortly after your treatment ends. Others may persist for years before resolving, and some may never go away completely. There are also late effects associated with treatment— effects that can appear up to years following cessation of treatment. It helps to be aware of these long-term and late effects so that you can incorporate this information into your treatment decisions. It is also important that you bring up these issues with your doctor so that, if at all possible, steps can be taken to eliminate or ameliorate these treatment-related problems. As cancer patients are surviving longer, more is becoming known about these long-term health issues. This increased awareness helps patients to recognize these effects, and seek treatment and/or proper follow-up care. Advances in cancer care are also bringing about more effective treatments with less adverse effects.

The following is a list of some of the long-term and late effects associated with standard lung cancer treatments. Keep in mind that some patients do not experience any long-term problems stemming from their treatment, although it is more common that you will have some residual effects. If you experience chronic long-term pain as a result of your cancer treatment, you should not "learn to live with it"—ask your doctor for a referral to a pain clinic.

- **Surgery.** Depending on the extent of your surgery, you will likely have reduced lung function, creating physical limitations. This function may improve over time as your remaining lung tissue expands, but it may never return to presurgery capacity. You may also have numbness and nerve pain at and around the surgical site. Other reported late effects include muscle and bone pain and heartburn/reflux, resulting from shifts in your musculo-skeletal system and esophagus following lung surgery.

- **Chemotherapy.** Peripheral neuropathy is a common long-term effect of cisplatin or Taxol chemotherapy (see Question 79). Hearing loss or ringing in the ears is experienced occasionally with high doses of cisplatin. Permanent damage to fertility is possible. Some patients also report a reduction in mental function ("fuzzy thinking" and problems with memory) that is frequently referred to as "chemo brain." It is not uncommon for patients to experience fatigue that persists long after chemotherapy has ended. Serious but relatively rare problems include kidney, lung, and heart damage as well as the increased risk of a second malignancy, such as leukemia.

- **Radiation Therapy.** Radiation to the chest can cause permanent scarring in the lungs (**radiation fibrosis**), thereby creating significant long-term breathing problems for some patients. In rare cases, patients can also experience damage to the heart or spine. These serious effects are becoming even less common as advances in technology enable far greater precision in delivering radiation to lung tumors while sparing healthy tissue.

Radiation fibrosis

scarring of the lungs caused by radiation treatment

Living with Lung Cancer

How should I change my diet following a lung cancer diagnosis? Should I take dietary supplements? Can diet affect my survival from lung cancer?

Is there any reason to quit smoking? How can I quit smoking while dealing with the stress of lung cancer?

More . . .

84. How should I change my diet following a lung cancer diagnosis? Should I take dietary supplements? Can diet affect my survival from lung cancer?

Many patients wonder whether there is anything they can do to alter their diet in order to influence the course of their disease. Frequently, patients will hear from friends and family that adopting certain dietary habits will make a critical difference in their survival: "drink tons of green tea, it will cure your disease," or "stay away from sugar, it will feed your tumor." Although studies have shown that people who consume diets high in fruits and vegetables have a lower risk of developing lung cancer, there is no conclusive evidence that specific dietary changes made after a diagnosis of lung cancer can affect long-term survival.

This does not mean there is no reason to pay attention to your diet. Eating a healthy diet is good for you and can only be beneficial when you are fighting a life-threatening disease. Eating affects how you feel, your energy level, and your overall health. The American Cancer Society's nutrition recommendations include: 1) Eat five or more servings of fruits and vegetables each day; 2) choose whole grains over processed (refined) grains and sugars; 3) limit consumption of red meats, particularly those high in fat and processed; and 4) limit consumption of alcoholic beverages, if you drink at all.[3] Of course, if you are

---

[3]American Cancer Society. (2001). ACS Recommendations for Nutrition and Physical Activity for Cancer Prevention. (*www.cancer.org*)

suffering from cancer or treatment-induced weight loss, then you have special dietary needs and your doctor will advise you on what you can do to gain weight (see Question 82).

There is similarly no definitive evidence that dietary supplementation can affect your lung cancer. If you do choose to take supplements, alert your doctor so that he or she can advise you as to whether the supplements might interfere with your cancer treatments. It is a good idea to take a multivitamin to ensure you are getting your minimum daily requirements of vitamins and minerals necessary for good health.

85. Is there any reason to quit smoking? How can I quit smoking while dealing with the stress of lung cancer?

Yes, there are strong and compelling reasons to quit smoking following a lung cancer diagnosis. The National Cancer Institute has found that cancer patients who continue to smoke may reduce the effectiveness of their treatment and increase the likelihood of a second cancer. There is also reason to believe that continued smoking may worsen the side effects of treatment, put you at increased risk for complications following lung surgery, and decrease your survival time. One study conducted in small cell lung cancer patients found that survival correlated with smoking status: the patients who continued to smoke after their diagnosis had the poorest survival; the patients who quit at diagnosis fared better; and the patients who had quit on average 2.5 years prior to diagnosis survived the longest.[4]

---

[4]National Cancer Institute. (2001). PDQ: Smoking Cessation and Continued Risk in Cancer Patients. (*www.cancer.gov*)

Consider how the following health benefits of smoking cessation might affect you at this critical time in your life:

- Your circulation will improve.
- Your pulse rate and blood pressure, which are abnormally high while smoking, will return to normal.
- Your sense of taste and smell will return.
- Your breathing will become easier.
- Your risk of developing infections such as pneumonia (a common cause of death in people with lung cancer) is reduced.
- Your risk of developing other smoking-related disease, including heart disease and lung disease, are reduced.[5]

It is never too late to quit.

It is never too late to quit. Even following your lung cancer diagnosis, smoking cessation will have a positive impact on your health, your quality of life and, possibly, your survival.

Your challenge is to motivate yourself to quit smoking during an extremely stressful time in your life. For some people this is easy—just hearing the words "lung cancer" is sufficient motivation. For others, the quitting process becomes even more difficult because smoking relieves the anxiety that comes with having lung cancer. Although quitting smoking is hard work, there are proven methods available to help you. The Surgeon General recommends **nicotine replacement therapy** (in patch, gum, inhaler, and nasal spray forms)

Nicotine replacement therapy

smoking cessation method that uses nicotine substitutes in various forms, including a patch, gum, inhaler, or nasal spray

[5]National Cancer Institute. (2000). Cancer Facts: Questions and Answers About Smoking Cessation. (*www.cancer.gov*)

and the antidepressant, Bupropion, as reliable drug treatments that increase long-term quit rates. The effectiveness of these drugs is further increased with counseling, including behavior modification therapy, problem-solving/skills training, and social support. The more intense the counseling, the more likely you are to quit.[6]

Your doctor can help you to find the combination of cessation methods that will work best for you and advise you on smoking cessation programs that are available in your community. Remember that you may have to make several attempts before you succeed—don't get discouraged. Keep trying and don't try to go it alone—seek support when you need it. For information on organizations, programs, and Internet resources to help you stop smoking, see Question 100.

Not everyone who is diagnosed with lung cancer is able to quit smoking. Although there are unequivocal health benefits, there are also understandable reasons why it is not possible for some patients with advanced lung cancer to quit. In those cases, it is important for the patient and the patient's family to let go of any guilt or anger over smoking. Conflict over smoking only serves to layer additional stress on top of an already stressful existence. If you or your family cannot come to terms with your continued smoking, you should seek professional counseling to resolve this divisive issue.

Remember that you may have to make several attempts before you succeed—don't get discouraged.

---

[6]U.S. Public Health Service. Treating Tobacco Use and Dependence. Summary. (*www.surgeongeneral.gov/tobacco/smokesum.htm*)

Living with Lung Cancer

86. What are the benefits of exercise for lung cancer patients?

Exercise can improve both your physical and mental health. It is no different when you have lung cancer. The general benefits ascribed to exercise—increased strength and energy, elevated mood—are even more desirable when you are battling cancer. The problem is that both your cancer and its treatment make exercise a more difficult prospect. However, studies in breast cancer patients have demonstrated that a 20 to 30 minute walking program (5 to 6 times per week) during chemotherapy or radiation therapy helps to decrease levels of fatigue and emotional distress, and increase sleep quality, physical functioning, and quality of life.[7] In some cases, exercise can provide both relief and distraction. So there are compelling reasons to get out of your chair and walk—even if it's just a few more steps than yesterday.

A useful exercise for lung cancer patients to learn is called abdominal breathing. Abdominal breathing can help to expand your lungs and increase the flow of oxygen. This is especially desirable for patients who have had surgery to remove a portion of their lung(s). Pulmonary therapists can teach you abdominal breathing and provide additional exercises to maximize your breathing capacity. Physical therapists can show you exercises to increase your upper body strength and range of motion. These exercises are not just for rehabilitation; they can help you over the long term to weather the physical changes that result from surgery.

---

[7]Clark, Patricia M. (2001). Exercise in Cancer-Related Fatigue Management. *26th Congress of the Oncology Nursing Society*. Medscape Conference Coverage. (*www.medscape.com*)

If your surgeon has not given you a referral to a physical therapist, ask for one.

87. What should I know about stress and the immune system? How does stress affect my survival and my ability to cope with my disease? Can complementary therapies help to reduce my stress?

A lung cancer diagnosis brings a pile of additional stress into your life: the stress of knowing you have a life-threatening disease; the stress of deciding what treatment to pursue; the stress of the treatment itself; the stress brought on by the impact of your cancer on the lives of your family and on your daily routine; the stress of explaining your lung cancer to your family and friends (and of dealing with their reactions); the stress of how your lung cancer affects your ability to work and your financial situation—the list of cancer-related stressors is seemingly endless. Stress is an undesirable condition that can adversely affect both your physical and mental well-being. Stress can compromise your immune system and take away your ability to relax and seek peace of mind. Although there is no evidence that stress will cause your tumor to grow faster or lessen your chances for long-term survival, it makes sense that someone who is highly stressed experiences a reduced quality of life.

The first step in reducing the stress in your life is to identify your stressors. Make a list of everything you can think of that provokes anxiety or causes you to feel additional stress, whether cancer-related or not. Take time to think about how you can eliminate these stressors from your life or reduce the negative impact they have on you. Be creative. Delegate whenever possible.

Don't be shy about asking for help or backing out of commitments made prior to your diagnosis. People will understand that lung cancer has changed your priorities and that you now have to focus on your health. Don't be tied to activities that have more of a negative effect on your life than a positive effect. You'll be amazed at how much stress you can eliminate when you sit down and take stock of the nonessentials in your life.

The ultimate challenge for most patients, however, is the stress brought on by family and financial obligations, and by the physical and emotional consequences of having lung cancer. If your ability to cope with these responsibilities interferes with your daily functioning, you should seek professional counseling. There are also complementary therapies that can help you to manage your stress. If you can find activities that help you to relax and feel less stressed, you will be better able to cope with the challenges that come your way. Complementary therapies that are used by cancer patients to reduce stress include relaxation and meditation, exercise programs such as yoga and tai chi, hypnotherapy, biofeedback, massage, and art and music therapy. Many cancer centers offer these types of therapies to patients. For further information on complementary therapies, see Question 100.

88. What about returning to work? I am worried about being able to function at 100 percent. What are my rights?

Returning to work after time off for cancer treatment can be both a physical and psychological challenge. You may have physical limitations as a result of your treatment, such as breathing problems and fatigue, which make full time employment difficult. You may also worry about the reactions of your co-workers to your cancer and dread answering their questions about your health. The process of returning to work is different for everyone. Whether it will be a smooth transition for you depends on a number of factors: the extent of your physical limitations; your comfort level in sharing information about your cancer with your coworkers; how supportive (and flexible) your employer is about your needs; your attitude toward your work; and the physical and emotional demands of your job.

Before you negotiate the terms of your return to work, it is important that you are aware of your rights and protections under both federal and state law. The Americans with Disabilities Act (ADA) prohibits discrimination by both public and private employers against qualified workers with disabilities or histories of disabilities. The Federal Rehabilitation Act of 1973 ensures that federal employers or companies receiving federal funds cannot discriminate against cancer survivors (among others) in hiring practices, promotions, transfers, and layoffs at the federal level. You may have additional employment protections depending upon the laws in your state.

It is important that you are aware of your rights and protections under both federal and state law.

Planning for your return to work can make a difference: know your rights, consider how you will respond to questions from coworkers, and think ahead about what accommodations you might require on a short- or long-term basis so that you will be prepared to discuss your options with your employer. See Question 100 for resources that can assist you in determining your employment rights as a cancer survivor, provide information on how to ease your transition back to work, and direct you to resources you can turn to in the event that you suffer workplace discrimination.

89. What happens when my treatment ends? Why don't I feel happy—or at least relieved?

If your treatment has been successful, and there is no evidence of your lung cancer, you have reason to celebrate. Your hopes for long-term survival, and for a normal life with your friends and family, are closer to becoming a reality. Yet, while you may feel happy on one level, you may also feel distressed on another. This emotional conflict is not unusual. With lung cancer, the fear of recurrence is ever-present. Active treatment may have given you a sense of security; however, now that your treatment has stopped, your level of anxiety may have increased. You may feel somewhat abandoned—most likely you have become used to frequent office or hospital visits, and have developed close relationships with your doctors, nurses, and the receptionists, and now you are not going to see them for awhile. You may also be coping with treatment-related side effects—breathing issues, fatigue, peripheral neuropathy—that interfere with daily life. Your support system may disappear when your treatment ends. Family and friends may hear your good news and stop inquiring after you—the cards, e-mails, phone calls, and visits that had uplifted you in the past may become less frequent or cease entirely. This is a time of transition. It is not surprising that many lung cancer survivors find it difficult to finish treatment and carry on with their lives.

Many lung cancer survivors find it difficult to finish treatment and carry on with their lives.

A lung cancer support group may be helpful to you at this time (see Question 24). Here, you may find other lung cancer survivors who are facing similar circumstances. You will also be able to reach out to newly diagnosed patients. This effort to help others can make you feel good about yourself and remind you about how far you have come. If your anxiety causes you to feel depressed or interferes with your functioning, you should talk to your doctor and ask whether counseling or medication might help to alleviate your distress. You should also let your family and friends know that you still need their support even though you are no longer in treatment. They may assume everything is OK unless you take the time to explain your ongoing needs.

The most important thing you can do during this time is to be vigilant about your follow-up care. Although follow-up care for lung cancer varies among doctors, you should be aware and comfortable with your doctor's recommendations for office visits, blood tests, and scans. If you are worried about recurrence, ask your doctor if there are any chemoprevention trials that might be appropriate for you (see Question 96). In addition to your lung cancer-related concerns, you should discuss "well care" with your doctor. It is important that you take good care of your health (good nutrition, exercise) so that you can be strong in your survival.

What will be most effective for resolving your emotional distress, and sometimes also your treatment side effects, is the passage of time. As each day passes, you will feel more comfortable with your status as a lung cancer survivor. You will adjust to the emotional, physical, and social changes brought about by your lung cancer experience and find a new equilibrium—a new normal—that will carry you through your life.

90. What about follow-up care? How often should I be seen? What is my doctor looking for?

After you have completed treatment for your lung cancer, it is important that you receive regular follow-up care. Your doctor will want to see you to check for recurrence of your lung cancer, to manage any long-term effects from your cancer and its treatment, and to monitor for a second lung cancer or other primary cancer.

The American Society of Clinical Oncologists (ASCO) recommends the following follow-up schedule for asymptomatic lung cancer patients treated with curative intent: every 3 months during the first 2 years; every 6 months during years 3 through 5; and yearly thereafter. More frequent visits may be warranted if a patient experiences symptoms or has coexisting conditions that require closer surveillance.[8]

At each follow-up visit, your doctor will order certain blood tests, take a medical history, and perform a physical exam. X-rays and CT scans will be ordered regularly to monitor for recurrence in the lungs. Unfortunately, there are no standard recommendations for the frequency of these imaging studies, and practices among lung specialists vary widely. Although the brain and bone are common sites of metastasis in lung cancer, scans to detect metastatic disease (such as a

---

[8]ASCO. (2000). A Patient's Guide: Advanced Lung Cancer Treatment. (*www.asco.org/people/rs/html/m_patguidelung.htm*)

brain MRI or a bone scan) are usually ordered only if symptoms are present.

The purpose of follow-up care, however, is to detect recurrence or disease at an early stage when it can be treated curatively or, if that is not possible, to begin palliative treatment in a timely manner. You will want to ask your doctor what symptoms you should be concerned about and under what circumstances you should report them.

Even though you are at high risk of recurrence during the first few years after your diagnosis, your risk declines as time goes on. You remain at increased risk, however, for a second primary lung cancer, and surveillance for a second primary is critical because there is evidence that, when feasible, resection of second primaries can be very successful.

Although your primary concern during your follow-up visits will undoubtedly be to seek reassurance that your lung cancer has not recurred or that a second lung cancer has not developed, you should not hesitate to bring up ongoing health issues that impact your quality of life. It is not unusual for patients to experience depression following cessation of active treatment, and you should discuss this possibility with your doctor if you feel depressed or overly anxious and think you might benefit from counseling. Patients who have undergone chemotherapy, radiation, or surgery often experience long-term adverse effects that should be discussed on a regular basis so they can be properly addressed. (See Question 83 for discussion of long-term and late effects.) Do not feel that your complaints about ongoing treatment effects are too minor to bring up during

Living with Lung Cancer

Ask your doctor what symptoms you should be concerned about.

your follow-up visits. Your quality of life is important and your doctor should work with you to address these legitimate concerns.

91. Should I get a flu shot? What about the pneumonia vaccine?

Lung infections can pose a serious and potentially deadly threat to lung cancer patients. Safe and effective vaccines are available for both influenza (the flu) and pneumococcal pneumonia, two common lung infections. Note that these vaccines protect against two very specific diseases—influenza and pneumococcal pneumonia—and therefore are not a guarantee you will not contract another respiratory illness, such as the common cold. The flu shot is administered yearly, most optimally in October or November. You can get the pneumonia vaccine at any time, and revaccination is recommended after 5 years. Don't wait to ask your doctor about getting vaccinated; it could save your life.

If Treatment Fails

How do I decide if it's time to stop treatment?

What is hospice?

What can I do to prepare for my death?

More . . .

92. How do I decide when it's time to stop treatment?

Deciding when to stop treatment is an extremely difficult and personal decision that no one can make for you. Each person must come to this point on his or her own terms—there is no one way for you to decide. Often decisions to stop treatment come about when quality of life has become intolerable and there is no reason to expect that further treatment will be beneficial. However, this decision is deeply personal and can result from a confluence of circumstances. Most importantly, it should be based on your values and beliefs. You may seek counsel from the people who have helped you to make decisions along the way—this may include family members, friends, healthcare providers, spiritual advisors, and others. Family members and friends may provide guidance and support as you struggle with your decision, but you should realize that their counsel will be charged with their own emotions and views. This may create conflict and make the decision more difficult for you. They may not be "ready." On the other hand, you may find that the view of your family is in line with yours, thereby making your decision easier. Ultimately, however, it is your decision to make. There is no way to predict how you will come to a decision to stop treatment and how others will react to your decision. What matters most is that you are at peace with the decision you have made.

Hospice

a concept of end-of-life care that focuses on palliative rather than curative care and provides comprehensive support to dying patients and their families

93. What is hospice?

Hospice is a concept of end-of-life care. Hospice care addresses quality-of-life concerns and provides palliative rather than curative care to dying patients (see Question 32). Hospice patients are cared for by a multidisciplinary team that may include doctors, nurses, nursing assistants, social workers, therapists, spiritual advisors, counselors, and hospice volunteers, among others. Hospice care provides comprehensive support to the terminally ill by addressing their medical, emotional, spiritual, and practical needs as well as by providing support for family members.

A primary focus of hospice care is to provide symptom relief, and hospice professionals are particularly expert at pain management. Many patients choose hospice care to ensure that their final days will be as pain-free as possible. Some hospices allow chemotherapy, providing it is given for palliative purposes; most hospices allow radiotherapy for the same reason.

Most often, hospice care is provided at home, but it is also offered in hospice centers or long-term care facilities. It is available to patients who have a terminal illness and who are no longer seeking curative treatment—this typically refers to patients with a life expectancy of 6 months or less. The range and amount of hospice services available to you will depend on your local hospice and on your insurance plan. Hospice coverage is provided by Medicare, and often also by Medicaid and private insurance providers. For further information on hospice and how to locate hospice services, see the resources listed in Question 100.

94. What can I do to prepare for my death?

Amid agonizing emotions and physical challenges, patients who are dying have decisions to make. Addressing these end-of-life issues proactively can help terminally-ill patients to resolve physical, psychological, and practical challenges in a manner consistent with personal beliefs, thereby providing some measure of comfort and peace of mind to both patient and family.

End-of-life medical care. Talk to your doctor about his or her comfort level in handling end-of-life issues. If he or she is not comfortable in handling these issues, or has done so only rarely, you might want to seek a palliative care consultation. A palliative care doctor specializes in the needs of terminally ill patients. You deserve to have symptom management and relief from pain during your final days, and you may want to consider hospice care at this time (see Question 93). It is critical that you communicate your wishes about your medical care at the end of life to your healthcare providers. **Advanced directives** will allow you to prepare for the medical possibilities and assign someone who can act on your behalf should you become unable to direct your own medical care (see Question 95). Your views on what "quality of life" and "death with dignity" mean to you are appropriate topics to discuss with both your doctors and healthcare proxy.

Think about your emotional and spiritual needs. Fear or denial of impending death, or anxiety about the dying process, is common. You may want to find someone with whom you can discuss your feelings about death and dying. This could be your doctor, your religious leader, a family member, or a close friend. Many patients also explore the meaning of their lives and of their cancer experiences during this time. This spiritual journey is important to patients, whether or not they are religious in any traditional sense.

Advanced directives

legal documents that allow you to prepare for future medical possibilities and to assign someone to act on your behalf in the event you become unable to direct your own medical care

You may want to find some- one with whom you can discuss your feelings about death and dying.

Take care of financial affairs, including making sure your will is in order. Though it is difficult to deal with these sensitive concerns, it will alleviate added burdens on your family after your death.

Attend to unfinished business—settle up emotional accounts. Make amends; say your goodbyes. Spend time with those who mean the most to you.

A palliative care specialist, your doctor, or a social worker will be able to refer you to end-of-life support resources. By preparing for the eventuality of death, you will help yourself and your family to cope with the dying process. Many terminally ill patients worry that they will be a burden to their families. This is less likely to occur when you have addressed these issues ahead of time: you'll have the satisfaction and peace of mind of knowing that you have done all you can to spare your family additional stress. You can then concentrate on your quality of life and on sharing time with your loved ones during your final days.

95. What are advanced directives?

Advanced directives are legal documents that specify your wishes regarding your future medical care. They are used in the event that you become unable to make these decisions yourself. As a patient, you have the right to accept or refuse medical treatment; advanced directives protect this right should you become incapacitated.

There are three types of advanced directives with which you should familiarize yourself:

Do Not Resuscitate (DNR) order. Your doctor may (in fact, should) ask you about a DNR order. This may be a very uncomfortable subject to discuss, but it is something everyone should think about, regardless of one's health. Your doctor wants to know whether, in the event of a cardiac or respiratory arrest (e.g., a massive heart attack or if you stop breathing, regardless of the reason), you would want "heroic" measures performed—that is, whether you would want doctors to do whatever is necessary to keep you alive. These measures could involve shocking your chest, putting in a breathing tube, or putting you on a ventilator (breathing machine) in the intensive care unit. Some considerations to keep in mind before you decide:

- How strong are you? Very weak patients rarely recover enough to eventually get off the breathing machine and leave the intensive care unit, regardless of what caused their heart or lungs to stop.
- Why did this happen? If it happened because of a complication of the lung cancer, and if the lung cancer is advanced and unlikely to be controlled, the chances of successfully coming off the ventilator are very remote.
- How difficult will it be for your family to face making the decision as to when it is extremely unlikely you will be able to get off the ventilator, and when to stop trying? (The horrible euphemism is "When to pull the plug?")

There are several reasons why it is very important that you think about this issue and discuss it with your family *before* you get seriously ill:

- It is much easier to be calm and objective when talking about a "hypothetical" event.

- Very often, the heart or lungs can stop working suddenly and there is not time to have a discussion as to whether to try to revive the patient. If a DNR order has not been written, the patient will almost always be "coded," and an attempt to resuscitate the patient will be made.

This is the one type of advanced directive that does not require your signature—your doctor can write an order on your chart after having discussed it with you. Also, should you decide to be "DNR," ask your doctor or nurse about a DNR bracelet. This is a small plastic band, similar to a hospital identification band, worn around the wrist, that indicates you do not want to be resuscitated in the event of a cardiac or respiratory arrest. This bracelet will prevent paramedics from trying to resuscitate you should you collapse out in public.

Living will. A living will specifies which medical treatments you do and do not want to have should you become unable to decide for yourself. It is important that you discuss your living will with your doctor. Your doctor can explain any medical and ethical details that you need to know in order to make decisions about end-of-life care. The National Cancer Institute recommends that you consider the following life-sustaining measures when drawing up your living will:

- the use of life-sustaining equipment (dialysis machines, ventilators, and respirators)
- "do not resuscitate" (DNR) orders; artificial hydration and nutrition (tube feeding)
- withholding of food and fluids

- palliative/comfort care
- organ and tissue donation[9]

A critical part of the living will process is to discuss your wishes with your family and loved ones. This will allow them to more easily understand and accept your decisions.

Durable power of attorney for health care. A durable power of attorney for health care is also known as a medical power of attorney. This type of advanced directive allows you to specify a healthcare proxy—a trusted person such as your spouse or other loved one—to make medical decisions for you should you become unable to do so for yourself. You should share your general and specific views regarding life-sustaining care and end-of-life issues with the person who will be your healthcare proxy, and make sure this person will be able to make your medical decisions for you—even under circumstances in which your wishes may not be known.

Most hospitals, lawyers, and palliative care physicians recommend a durable power of attorney over a living will, because a living will can never foresee all possibilities as to what may happen to a person. If you have designated a power of attorney, however, and this person knows you well, he or she probably will know what you would want done regardless of the circumstance.

An excellent source for additional information on advanced directives is Partnership for Caring

---

[9]National Cancer Institute. (2000). Cancer Facts: Advanced Directives. (*www.cancer.gov*)

(*www.partnershipforcaring.org*). Partnership for Caring provides state-specific advance directive packages that can be downloaded from its web site or ordered by phone at 800–989–9455 or 410–962–5454. Copies of your executed documents should be given to your doctor and your healthcare proxy.

You shouldn't worry that by preparing an advanced directive, you are giving up on your hope for survival or turning your lung cancer into an automatic death sentence. Ideally, everyone should have advanced directives—not just people with serious or life-threatening conditions. By grappling with these difficult end-of-life issues ahead of time, and by discussing them with your family and loved ones, you will have removed a potential source of distress for them and given yourself peace of mind that your wishes will be carried out.

If Treatment Fails

Prevention, Screening, and Advocacy

Can lung cancer be prevented?

What is chemoprevention?

Is there a screening test for lung cancer?

More . . .

96. Can lung cancer be prevented? What is chemoprevention?

The key to preventing lung cancer is smoking prevention and cessation.

The key to preventing lung cancer is smoking prevention and cessation. Active smoking is responsible for 85–90% of all lung cancers, and exposure to second-hand smoke accounts for a significant portion of the remaining cases. Preventing people from smoking would result in a vast reduction in the incidence of lung cancer. Tragically, there has been little progress toward reaching this goal. Tobacco companies continue to be effective in marketing their deadly product to teenagers, who are likely to ignore the risks associated with smoking. Messages that promote smoking as a cool behavior permeate our culture, making a mockery of anti-smoking campaigns. Public health initiatives in smoking prevention have not succeeded—we need more, and more effective, school-based prevention programs beginning in preschool. And children and adults who are already smoking deserve better access to resources that will help them quit. Although smoking cessation will reduce the likelihood of getting lung cancer, a smoker's risk will never be equal to a non-smoker. The best advice to prevent lung cancer is to never start smoking, and to avoid chronic exposure to secondhand smoke.

Other environmental hazards, such as exposure to asbestos and radon, are responsible for a small percentage of lung cancer cases. Federal safety regulations are helping to prevent exposure to these and other lung carcinogens in the workplace.

Clinical trials are underway to determine whether lung cancer can be prevented in people who are at high risk for the disease, such as current and former smokers and people with a history of lung cancer. These studies are called chemoprevention trials. They are designed to test whether natural or chemical substances can prevent cancer.

Findings from previous chemoprevention trials involving beta-carotene and alpha-tocopherol (a type of vitamin E) were discouraging. The results in some cases showed that these supplements actually increased the incidence of lung cancer in smokers. As more is learned about lung **carcinogenesis**, scientists continue to test promising chemopreventive agents, such as Iressa, Celebrex, and selenium. If your lung cancer is in remission, you may be a candidate for a chemoprevention trial. Ask your doctor whether this might be a good option for you. Because increased participation will help find ways to prevent lung cancer, you should encourage your family and friends who are current or former smokers to consider chemoprevention trials. For information on locating chemoprevention trials, see Question 100.

Carcinogenesis
the development of cancer

97. Is there a screening test for lung cancer?

It is important to first understand what a screening test is. A screening test looks at asymptomatic individuals with a particular risk factor for a disease in hopes of making an early diagnosis to improve survival. This is different from a diagnostic test, which is done to confirm the presence of a disease in a patient who already has symptoms. Currently there is no recommended screening test for lung cancer as exists for breast (mammography), colon (fecal occult blood and sigmoidoscopy), and prostate (prostate specific antigen

[PSA]) cancers. The lack of an effective screening program for lung cancer is devastating. Without screening, lung cancer patients do not get diagnosed until they become symptomatic—when, invariably, their cancer is advanced and incurable.

Lung cancer screening has long been mired in controversy. This is because although there are screening tests that have the potential to identify lung cancer in its early stages, there has been no scientific study that demonstrates that any of these tests can reduce mortality for lung cancer patients.

In the past, chest x-rays have been used for lung cancer screening on an informal basis, and there are lung cancer specialists who believe that chest x-rays done in high-risk populations find enough early cancers to justify their use as a screening test. However, most specialists feel that by the time a lung cancer has grown to the point that it can be seen on a chest x-ray, it may have already spread to other parts of the body. Randomized screening trials in the 1970s failed to show that smokers who underwent annual chest x-rays lived longer than those who did not; the American Cancer Society, which interprets available screening data, does not recommend a chest x-ray as a screening tool for lung cancer. However, there are some scientists who now say those studies were flawed, so the debate over x-ray screening for lung cancer continues.

A promising new technology called a low-dose spiral CT scan has been shown to be more sensitive at detecting small lung nodules than x-ray. It is not yet known whether detection of very small lung nodules will result in fewer lung cancer deaths, but trials are underway to test the usefulness of low-dose spiral CT scanning as a screening test in high-risk individuals. This test is similar to a diagnostic CT test, but its pictures are taken much more quickly and expose the patient to lower doses of radiation. The risks and benefits of this test are currently being hotly debated: even though lung cancers are found when they are smaller, is it still too late? Have they already spread? Also, it turns out that a large percentage of people have very small abnormalities on CT scans and, in most cases, it is unclear as to what these abnormalities are. Thus, many people need to be followed with repeat CT scans for years before the radiologist feels comfortable calling these abnormalities benign. The price of such screening tests may therefore be the cost to society of the intensive follow-up that most patients will have to undergo, as well as the anxiety these tests produce. There is a large clinical trial underway at many medical centers throughout the world to try to better understand whether this approach is likely to reduce the individual and societal burdens of lung cancer. Currently, most insurance companies are not paying for the screening CT.

If you have friends and family who are current or former smokers, you should make them aware of screening trials for lung cancer. Other candidates for screening include individuals who have had significant exposure to environmental carcinogens, such as second-hand smoke, radon, and asbestos (in the home or in the workplace) and individuals with a family history of lung cancer. For information on locating screening trials, see Question 100.

98. Does lung cancer run in families? Is my family at increased risk for lung cancer because I have lung cancer?

There are some families that have a high incidence of lung cancer. Scientists are studying these families to determine why certain people are at greater risk for developing this deadly disease. It is likely that blood relatives with lung cancer share genetic mutations (abnormalities) that make them more susceptible to smoking and other environmental carcinogens. This is probably due to the fact that some people metabolize (neutralize and excrete) carcinogens (cancer-causing substances) in cigarette smoke better than others. Several studies have shown that women may be more susceptible to developing lung cancer than men. Although our present understanding is limited, research into families with lung cancer is shedding light on the complex relationship among the lifestyle, environmental and genetic factors that comprise lung cancer risk.

Currently, there is no genetic test to determine risk for lung cancer. Thus, there is no way to know whether your family (particularly your siblings and children) may be at increased risk because of your lung cancer. As genetic markers for lung cancer risk continue to be identified and characterized, this may change. It makes sense for anyone with a family history of lung cancer to discuss this, and other risk factors, with his or her doctor. There are no recommendations for widespread screening for lung cancer, although a doctor may choose to increase surveillance for individuals in certain cases.

If two or more members of your family have lung cancer, you may be able to participate in a family research study. For more information, contact the Johns Hopkins National Familial Lung Cancer Registry by phone at 410–614–1910 or visit its web site at *www.path.jhu.edu/nfltr.html.*

99. Why has there been so little progress in fighting lung cancer? What can I do to help?

It is dispiriting and frustrating to learn that although lung cancer is the number one cancer killer of men and women, it is funded at significantly lower levels than the other common cancers. Lung cancer advocates have long argued that this disparity exists because lung cancer is associated with smoking and perceived by the public as a self-inflicted disease. This smoking stigma affects both public support and media coverage of lung cancer. It also affects the willingness of people with lung cancer to stand up and speak out about this deadly disease. Many lung cancer survivors feel guilty about their smoking and fear public scorn if they were to demand more dollars for lung cancer research. And, for many people with lung cancer, the possibility of becoming an advocate is out of the question—the sad fact is that the overwhelming majority of people with lung cancer will not survive their disease. They are too sick to advocate for themselves. In addition, although there are numerous advocacy organizations for breast, colon and prostate cancers, the Alliance for Lung Cancer Advocacy, Support, and Education (ALCASE) is the sole organization dedicated to lung cancer.

Nevertheless, there is reason to believe that the outlook is changing for people with lung cancer. In 2001, the National Cancer Institute (NCI) held an important meeting called the Lung Cancer Progress Review

Group (PRG) Roundtable that brought together over 100 leading scientists and clinicians along with several lung cancer advocates. The meeting resulted in a comprehensive report that put forth a national agenda for lung cancer research. In addition to identifying scientific goals and challenges, the report specifically addresses the issues of disproportionate funding and stigma ("blame the victim") as barriers to progress. You can obtain the Lung Cancer PRG report by calling 1–800–4-CANCER, or by visiting the online report: *prg.nci.nih.gov/lung/finalreport.html.*

There are countless ways that individuals can help to effect the changes necessary to make this PRG "strategy for progress" a reality. Here are a few places to start:

Familiarize yourself with the issues. Read the Lung Cancer PRG Report. Read the lung cancer information on the NCI's web site, *www.cancer.gov.* Read everything on lung cancer that you come across in the media. Think about how these issues affect you, and how they affect other lung cancer survivors, as well as people at risk for lung cancer.

Contact ALCASE. Let ALCASE know you are interested in participating in advocacy activities. ALCASE sponsors and coordinates efforts to influence policy and funding for lung cancer research, to raise awareness of lung cancer, and to increase support services for people with lung cancer.

Let your voice be heard. Write to your representatives in Washington and to your local media about lung cancer and lung cancer issues. Volunteer to participate in school anti-smoking programs. Visit local hospitals and advocate for increased information and support services for lung cancer patients. ALCASE can provide guidance and materials for your advocacy efforts and connect you with other survivors who are interested in effecting change. Remember, there is strength in numbers. Lung cancer advocates are working hard to network with each other and to emulate the progress that has come about for breast, prostate, and colon cancers. Our voices are gradually becoming a chorus.

Put a face on lung cancer. You do not have to become a full-time advocate to make a difference in the fight against lung cancer. Each time you identify yourself as a lung cancer survivor, you are putting a face on lung cancer. You are telling the world that people with lung cancer matter and deserve the same respect as people with other forms of cancer. You are bringing others into the lung cancer community. This is a battle we all can win together.

100. Where can I find more information about lung cancer?

The Appendix that follows is a selection of good resources for lung cancer patients and their families.

Cancer/Lung Cancer Information

Alliance for Lung Cancer Advocacy, Support and Education (ALCASE)
P.O. Box 849, Vancouver, WA 98666
Phone: 360–696–2436 or 800–298–2436
Web site: *www.alcase.org*
ALCASE is the only nonprofit organization dedicated solely to supporting and improving the quality of lives of people with lung cancer. ALCASE should be your first source for information and support following a lung cancer diagnosis.

American Cancer Society
National Home Office, 1599 Clifton Road, Atlanta, GA 30329
Phone: 800-ACS–2345
Web site: *www.cancer.org*
ACS is a nationwide, community-based organization that conducts cancer advocacy and research activities and provides patient education and support services. Information available in Spanish.

American Lung Association
1740 Broadway, New York, NY 10019
Phone: 212–315–8700
Web site: *www.lungusa.org*
The mission of ALA is to prevent lung disease and promote lung health, with special emphasis on asthma, tobacco control and environmental health. Information available in Spanish.

American Society of Clinical Oncology (ASCO)
1900 Duke Street, Suite 200
Alexandria, VA 22314
Phone: 703-299-0150
Web site: *www.asco.org*
ASCO is a professional organization for cancer specialists. New findings in cancer research are presented each year at its annual conference. Conference abstracts are posted on the ASCO web site.

Lung Cancer Online

Web site: *www.lungcanceronline.org*

Comprehensive directory to lung cancer information and
resources for patients and their families. Edited by Karen Parles.

Lungcancer.org

Web site: *www.lungcancer.org*

Lung cancer information for patients, healthcare professionals
and the media. Sponsored by Cancer Care and the Oncology
Nursing Society.

National Cancer Institute (NCI)

Public Inquiries Office, Building 31, Room 10A31, Bethesda,
MD 20892–2580

Phone: 800–4CANCER (NCI's Cancer Information Service)

Web site: *www.cancer.gov*

The NCI offers extensive up-to-date online and print information on lung cancer and its treatment, including clinical trials.
Information available in Spanish.

People Living with Cancer

Web site: *www.plwc.org*

Oncologist-approved information for people with cancer.
Maintained by ASCO.

Steve Dunn's Cancerguide

Web site: *cancerguide.org*

Steve Dunn, a kidney cancer survivor, provides a patient's perspective and valuable advice on how to find the answers to your
questions about cancer and most importantly, how to know
which questions to ask.

Print Publications

ALCASE publications include a lung cancer manual, and
newsletters for patients ("Spirit and Breath") and physicians
("Quarterly Scan").

Henschke, Claudia, et al. *Lung Cancer: Myths, Facts, Choices—
and Hope*. New York: W. W. Norton, 2002.

*InTouch Magazine: The Good Health Guide to Cancer Prevention
and Treatment*. Subscription available by phone at
877–246–8682 or online at *www.intouchlive.com*

Johnston, Lorraine. *Lung Cancer: Making Sense of Diagnosis, Treatment & Options*. Sebastopol, CA: O'Reilly & Associates, 2001.

Caregivers & Home Care

Family Caregiver Alliance
690 Market Street, Suite 600, San Francisco, CA 94104
Phone: 415–434–3388
Web site: *www.caregiver.org*
Caregiver resources include an online support group and an
information clearinghouse. Information available in Spanish.

National Family Caregivers Association
10400 Connecticut Avenue, #500, Kensington, MD 20895–3944
Phone: 800–896–3650
Web site: *www.nfcacares.org*
Provides education, information, support and advocacy services
for family caregivers.

CAREGIVERS (Association of Cancer Online Resources)
Web page: *www.acor.org Click on "Mailing Lists" and then select
"CAREGIVERS."*
Online discussion group for caregivers of cancer patients.

**Caring for the Caregiver (National Coalition for Cancer
Survivorship)**
Web page: *www.cansearch.org/programs/Caregiver.PDF*

**Guide for Cancer Supporters: Step-by-Step Ways to Help a
Relative or Friend Fight Cancer (R.A. Bloch Cancer
Foundation)**
Web page: *www.blochcancer.org/guide/guidechp1.html*

Print Publications
Houts, Peter S. and Julia A. Bucher, eds. *Caregiving: A Step-by-Step
Resource for Caring for the Person with Cancer at Home.* Atlanta,
GA: American Cancer Society, 2000.

Children

Kids Konnected
27071 Cabot Road, Suite 102, Laguna Hills, CA 92653
Phone: 949–582–5443
Web site: *www.kidskonnected.org*
Provides extensive support resources and programs for children
who have a parent with cancer.

What Do I Tell the Children? — A Guide for a Parent with Cancer (CancerBACUP)
Web page: *www.cancerbacup.org.uk/info/talk-children.htm*

Print Publications
Ackerman, Abigail and Adrienne Ackerman. *Our Mom Has Cancer*. Atlanta, GA: American Cancer Society, 2000.
Harpham, Wendy S. *When a Parent Has Cancer: A Guide to Caring for Your Children*. Companion book: *Becky and the Worry Cup*. New York: HarperCollins, 1997.

Clinical Trials Resources

There is no single resource for locating clinical trials for lung cancer. It makes sense to check all of the resources listed below repeatedly because new trials are continually added. There are also clinical trials services emerging that help to match patients to clinical trials. Some of these services can be useful for obtaining information and saving time, but it is important to read the company's privacy statement and know whether the company is being paid for recruiting patients before using them.

NCI Clinical Trials
Phone: 800–4CANCER
Web site: *www.cancer.gov/clinical_trials/*

The NCI offers comprehensive information on understanding and finding clinical trials, including access to the NCI/PDQ Clinical Trials Database.

NIH/NLM Clinical Trials
Web site: *ClinicalTrials.gov*
Clinical trials database service developed by the National Institute of Health's National Library of Medicine.

Centerwatch Clinical Trials Listing Service
Web site: *www.centerwatch.com*
Listing of clinical trials conducted by drug companies.

Clinical Trials Resources (Lung Cancer Online)

Web page: *www.lungcanceronline.org/clinical.htm*

In addition to linking to the major clinical trials resources listed above, Lung Cancer Online provides links to NCI-designated cancer centers and hospitals with lung cancer programs that are likely to be conducting clinical trials in lung cancer. These sites can be contacted directly for information on available lung cancer trials. Links to some clinical trials services can also be found in Lung Cancer Online's clinical trials section.

NCI Clinical Trials and Insurance Coverage

Web page:

cancertrials.nci.nih.gov/understanding/indepth/insurance/index.html

Excellent in-depth guide to clinical trials insurance issues.

Print Publications

Finn, Robert. *Cancer Clinical Trials: Experimental Treatments & How They Can Help You.* Sebastopol, CA: O'Reilly & Associates, 1999.

Mulay, Marilyn. *Making the Decision: A Cancer Patient's Guide to Clinical Trials.* Sudbury, MA: Jones & Bartlett Publishers, 2002.

Complementary and Alternative Medicine (CAM)

American Academy of Medical Acupuncture

Web site: *www.medicalacupuncture.org*

Professional site with articles on acupuncture, a list of frequently-asked-questions and acupuncturist locator.

Commonweal

P.O. Box 316, Bolinas, CA 94924

Phone: 415–868–0970

Web site: *www.commonweal.org*

Provides information on complementary approaches to cancer care, including the full-text of Michael Lerner's 1994 book, *Choices in Healing: Integrating the Best of Conventional and Complementary Approaches to Cancer*, published by MIT press (updated version available in print).

National Center for Complementary and Alternative Medicine (NCCAM)
Web site: *nccam.nih.gov*
Offers information on complementary and alternative medicine therapies, including NCI/PDQ expert-reviewed fact sheets on individual therapies and dietary supplements.

NCI Office of Cancer Complementary and Alternative Medicine (OCCAM)
Web site: *www3.cancer.gov/occam*
Information clearinghouse supporting the NCI's CAM activities.

Print Publications
American Cancer Society's Guide to Complementary and Alternative Cancer Methods. Atlanta, GA: American Cancer Society, 2000.
Benson, Herbert. *The Relaxation Response*. New York: Avon Books, 1975.
Cassileth, Barrie R. *The Alternative Medicine Handbook: The Complete Reference Guide to Alternative and Complementary Therapies*. New York: W.W. Norton & Company, 1998.
Kaptchuk, Ted. J. *The Web That Has No Weaver: Understanding Chinese Medicine*. McGraw-Hill, 2000.

Diet and Nutrition

American Institute for Cancer Research
1759 R Street, NW, Washington, DC 20009
Phone: 800–843–8114 202–328–7744 (in DC)
Web site: *www.aicr.org*
Supports research on diet and nutrition in the prevention and treatment of cancer. Provides information to cancer patients on nutrition and cancer, including a compilation of healthy recipes. Maintains a nutrition hotline for questions relating to nutrition and health.

Nutrition (American Cancer Society)
Web page: *www.cancer.org* (*Enter "nutrition" in the search box*).
Nutrition resources include: ACS guidelines on nutrition, dietary supplement information, nutrition message boards and tips on low-fat cooking and choosing healthy ingredients.

Drugs/Medications

MEDLINEplus: Drug Information
Web page: *www.medlineplus.gov (Click on the "drug information" button).*
A guide to over 9,000 prescription and over-the-counter medications provided by U.S. Pharmacopeia (USP).

Print Publications
Consumers Guide to Cancer Drugs. Atlanta, GA: American Cancer Society, 2000.

Employment, Insurance, Financial and Legal Resources

Americans with Disabilities Act (U.S. Department of Justice)
Web page: *www.usdoj.gov/crt/ada/adahom1.htm*

Cancer Legal Resource Center
919 S. Albany Street, Los Angeles, CA 90019-10015
Phone: 213–736–1455
A joint program of Loyola Law School and the Western Law Center for Disability Rights. Provides information and educational outreach on cancer-related legal issues to people with cancer and others impacted by the disease.

Centers for Medicare & Medicaid Services (CMS) (formerly the Health Care Financing Administration [HCFA])
Web site: *cms.hhs.gov*
Oversees administration of:
- **Medicare** – federal health insurance program for people 65 years or older and some disabled people under 65 years.
  Phone: 800–633–4227 Web site: *www.medicare.gov*
- **Medicaid** – federal and state health insurance program for certain low-income people. Contact your state Medicaid offices for further information.
  Web page: *www.hcfa.gov/medicaid/medicaid.htm*
- **Health Insurance Portability and Accountability Act (HIPAA)** – insurance reform that may lower your chance of losing existing coverage, ease your ability to switch health plans

and/or help you buy coverage on your own if you lose your employer's plan, and have no other coverage available.
Web page: *cms.hhs.gov Enter "HIPAA" in the search box.*

Family and Medical Leave Act (FMLA)
Web page: *www.dol.gov/dol/esa/fmla.htm*
U.S. Department of Labor web page providing information about the Family and Medical Leave Act (FMLA).

Health Insurance Association of America (HIAA)
1201 F Street, NW, Suite 500, Washington, DC 20004–1204
Phone: 202–824–1600
Web site: *www.hiaa.org/cons/cons.htm*
Provides insurance guides for consumers. Topics include health insurance and managed care, disability income, long-term care and medical savings accounts.

Hill-Burton Program (Health Resources and Services Administration)
Phone: 301–443–5656 800–638–0742 (800–492–0359 in Maryland)
Web page: *www.hrsa.gov:80/OSP/dfcr/obtain/obtain.htm*
Facilities that receive Hill-Burton funds from the government are required by law to provide services to some people who cannot afford to pay. Information on Hill-Burton eligibility and facilities locations is available via phone or Internet.

Patient Advocate Foundation
753 Thimble Shoals Boulevard, Suite B, Newport News, VA 23606
Phone: 800–532–5274
Web site: *www.patientadvocate.org*
Nonprofit organization helps patients to resolve insurance, debt and job discrimination matters relative to cancer. Patient resources include: *The National Financial Resources Guidebook for Patients: A State-by-State Directory, Your Guide to the Appeals Process and the Managed Care Answer Guide,* among others.

Social Security Administration (SSA)

Web site: *www.ssa.gov*

Oversees two programs that pay benefits to people with disabilities:

Social Security Disability Insurance – pays benefits to you and certain members of your family if you have worked long enough
and paid Social Security taxes

Supplemental Security Income – supplements Social Security pay-
ments based on need.

Veterans Health Administration

810 Vermont Avenue, NW, Washington, DC 20420

Phone: 202–273–5400 877–222–8387 (Health care benefits)

Web site: *www.va.gov/vbs/health/*

Eligible veterans and their dependents may receive cancer treatment
at a Veterans Administration Medical Center.

Print Publications

Hoffman, Barbara. *Working It Out: Your Employment Rights as a
Cancer Survivor.* Silver Spring, MD: National Coalition for
Cancer Survivorship, undated. This booklet can be ordered
from the NCCS at 877–622–7937.

Landry, David S. *Be Prepared: The Complete Financial, Legal and
Practical Guide to Living with Cancer, HIV and Other Life-Challenging Conditions.* New York: St. Martin's Press, 1998.

Financial Assistance Programs

Air Care Alliance

Phone: 888–260–9707

Web site: *www.aircareall.org*

Network of organizations willing to provide public benefit flights
for health care.

**Finding Ways to Pay for Care (National Coalition for Cancer
Survivorship)**

Web page: *www.cansearch.org. Select "Programs" and then "Cancer
Survival Toolbox"*

NeedyMeds
Web site: *www.needymeds.com*
Information on patient assistance programs and other programs
  that help people obtain medications, supplies and equipment.

Hospice & End-of-Life Issues

Partnership for Caring
1620 Eye Street, NW, Suite 202, Washington, DC 20006
Phone: 202–296–8071 800–989–9455
Web site: *www.partnershipforcaring.org*
Comprehensive information and resources covering end-of-life
  issues, including advanced directives.

**CANCER-HOSPICE (Association of Online Cancer
Resources)**
Web site: *www.acor.org Click on "Mailing Lists" and then select
  "CANCER-HOSPICE."*
Online discussion group for cancer patients dealing with hospice
  issues.

Growth House
Web site: *www.growthhouse.org*
Extensive, annotated directory to hospice and end-of-life
  resources. Organized by topic.

**Home Care Guide for Advanced Cancer (American College
of Physicians)**
Web page: *www.acponline.org/public/h_care/*
Guide for family and friends caring for advanced cancer patients
  who are living at home.

Hospice Net
Web site: *www.hospicenet.org*
Provides comprehensive information to patients and families facing
  life-threatening illness. Extensive resources addressing end-of-
  life issues from both patient and caregiver perspectives.

Patient Advocacy Skills

Cancer Survival Toolbox (National Coalition for Cancer Survivorship)
Web page: *www.cansearch.org Select "Programs" and then "Cancer Survival Toolbox."*
Topics include: communication skills, finding information, solving problems, making decisions, negotiating and standing up for your rights. (Also available as audiotapes at 877–866–5748.)

Information for the Asking: Questions to Help You Get the Information You Need from Your Healthcare Provider (ALCASE)
Web page: *www.alcase.org/publications/asking.html*

Print Publications
Anderson, Greg. *50 Essential Things to Do When the Doctor Says It's Cancer.* New York: Penguin Books, 1993.
Oster, Nancy et al. *Making Informed Medical Decisions: Where to Look and How to Use What You Find.* Sebastapol, CA: O'Reilly & Associates, Inc., 2000.
Willis, Joanie. *The Cancer Patient's Workbook.* New York: Dorling Kindersley Publishing, Inc., 2001.

Physician & Hospital Locators

American Society of Clinical Oncology (ASCO)
Web page: *www.asco.org Click on the "Find an Oncologist" button.*

American College of Surgeons (ACS) Commission on Cancer
Web page: *www.facs.org/public_info/yourhealth/aahcp.html*
Listing of ACS Commission on Cancer's Approved Hospital Cancer Programs.

American Medical Association (AMA) Physician Select
Web page: *www.ama-assn.org/aps/amahg.htm*
Provides professional information on licensed U.S. physicians.

Cardiothoracic Surgeons Network (CTSNet)
Web page: *www.ctsnet.org Click on the "Members" button.*
Database of cardiothoracic surgeons who are members of the
American Association of Thoracic Surgery (AATS), the Society
of Thoracic Surgeons (STS) or the European Association for
Cardio-Thoracic Surgery.

Lung Cancer Online: Lung Cancer Programs
Web page: *www.lungcanceronline.org/lcp*
Directory of institutions with multidisciplinary lung cancer pro-
grams, including NCI-designated cancer centers.

Prevention & Risk Assessment

Prevention (American Cancer Society)
Web page: *www.cancer.org. Enter "prevention" in the search box.*
Comprehensive section on prevention covers topics such as environmental and occupational cancer risks, exercise, tobacco and
cancer, nutrition for risk reduction and prevention and detection programs.

Your Cancer Risk (Harvard Center for Cancer Prevention)
Web site: *www.yourcancerrisk.harvard.edu*
Online lung cancer risk assessment tool.

Research Resources & Reference

PubMed: MEDLINE (National Library of Medicine)
Web site: *www.ncbi.nlm.nih.gov/PubMed/*
Provides free online access to MEDLINE, a database of over 11
million citations to the medical literature.

Medscape
Web site: *www.medscape.com. Enter "Lung Cancer Resource Center" in the search box.*
Medscape is an excellent source for latest news in lung cancer
research, including access to summaries of cancer conferences.
Aimed at health care professionals. Registration required for
free access to Medscape.

Merriam Webster Medical Dictionary
Web site: *www.intelihealth.com. Enter "Merriam Webster" in the search box.*
Registration required for free access to Intelihealth.

Print Publications
Laughlin, Edward H. *Coming to Terms with Cancer: A Glossary of Cancer-Related Terms* Atlanta, GA: American Cancer Society, 2002.

Smoking Cessation

Freedom from Smoking (American Lung Association)
Web page: *www.lungusa.org/ffs/*
Free online smoking cessation program designed to educate and modify smoking behavior patterns. This interactive course can be accessed 24 hours a day, 7 days a week.

Office of the Surgeon General: Tobacco Cessation
Web page: *www.surgeongeneral.gov/tobacco/default.htm*
See especially the "You Can Quit Smoking Consumer Guide." available by calling 202–401–4357.

Quitnet
Web site: *www.quitnet.org*
Comprehensive website for smoking cessation needs. Offers interactive personalized quitting tools, quitting guides, smoking cessation program locators, 24 hour online support/discussion, and links to smoking, tobacco and cessation-related information and resources.

Support Services

Alliance for Lung Cancer Advocacy, Support and Education (ALCASE)
P.O. Box 849, Vancouver, WA 98666
360–696–2436 800–298–2436
Web site: *www.alcase.org*
ALCASE offers a phone buddy program (individual patient-to-patient support) and maintains a geographic listing of in-person lung cancer support groups.

Association of Cancer Online Resources (ACOR)
Web site: *www.acor.org. Click on "Mailing Lists."*
ACOR offers online support groups for cancer patients. Lung cancer
lists include: a general list (LUNG-ONC), and specific lists for
small cell lung cancer (LUNG-SCLC), non-small cell lung cancer
(LUNG-NSCLC) and bronchioloalveolar (LUNG-BAC).

Cancer Care
275 Seventh Avenue, New York, NY 10001
Phone: 212–712–8080 800–813–4673
Web site: *www.cancercare.org*
Provides comprehensive support services and programs to peo-
ple with cancer.

Cancer Survivors Network
Web site: *www.acscsn.org*
ACSCSN is the American Cancer Society's online patient com-
munity.

R.A. Bloch National Cancer Foundation
4400 Main Street, Kansas City, MO 64111
Phone: 816–932–8453 800–433–0464
Web site: *www.blochcancer.org*
Provides Bloch-authored cancer books free of charge, a multidis-
ciplinary referral service and patient-to-patient phone support.

Vital Options International
15060 Ventura Boulevard, Suite 211, Sherman Oaks, CA 91403
Phone: 818–788–5225
Web site: *www.vitaloptions.org*
Produces "The Group Room," a weekly, syndicated radio call-in
show (with simultaneous webcast) covering important and
timely topics in cancer.

Wellness Community
35 East Seventh Street, Suite 412, Cincinnati, OH 45202
Phone: 513–421–7111 888–793-WELL
Web site: *www.wellness-community.org*
Provides educational programs and support groups for people
with cancer and their families.

Talking About Cancer (American Cancer Society)
Web page: *www.cancer.org. Enter "Talking About Cancer" in the
search box.*
Discusses how to talk about your cancer with family, friends, your
health care providers and your employer. Includes resources for
locating in-person and online support groups.

Print Publications
Coping with Cancer. Cancer magazine available free of charge in
oncology offices or by subscription at 615–791–3859 or
www.copingmag.com
Holland, Jimmie C. and Sheldon Lewis. *The Human Side of Cancer.*
New York: HarperCollins Publishers, 2000.
Schimmel, S.R., and Fox, B. *Cancer Talk: Voices of Hope and
Endurance from "The Group Room," the World's Largest Cancer Sup-
port Group.* New York: Broadway Books, 1999.

Symptoms, Side Effects & Complications

Fatigue
CancerFatigue.org
Web site: *www.cancerfatigue.org*
Information about cancer-related fatigue for patients and caregivers.

CANCER-FATIGUE (Association of Cancer Online Resources)
Web page: *www.acor.org Click on "Mailing Lists" and then select
"CANCER-FATIGUE."*
Online discussion list covering cancer and treatment-related fatigue.

**NCCN Cancer-Related Fatigue Treatment Guidelines for
Patients**
Web page: *www.nccn.org/patient_gls/_english/_fatigue/index.htm*

Print Publications
Harpham, Wendy S. "Resolving the Frustration of Fatigue." *CA:
A Cancer Journal for Clinicians.* 49 (1999): 178–189.
Outstanding article by a patient/physician discusses cancer-
related fatigue and how to deal with it.

Appendix

Nausea and Vomiting

NCCN Nausea and Vomiting Treatment Guidelines for Patients with Cancer

Web page: *www.nccn.org/patient_gls/_english/_nausea_and_vomiting/index.htm*

NCI/PDQ Nausea and Vomiting

Web page: *cancer.gov* Enter "nausea" in the search box.

Expert-reviewed information summary about cancer-related nausea and vomiting.

Nutritional Problems

NCI/PDQ Nutrition

Web site: *cancer.gov* Enter "nutrition" in the search box.

Expert-reviewed information summary about the causes and management of nutritional problems occurring in cancer patients.

Oral Complications

Oral Health, Cancer Care and You (National Institute of Dental and Craniofacial Research)

Web site: *nohic.aerie.com/campaign/*

NCI/PDQ Oral Complications of Chemotherapy and Head/Neck Radiation

Web page: *cancer.gov Enter "oral complications" in the search box.*

Pain

The National Pain Foundation (NPF)

P.O. Box 102605

Denver, CO 80250–2605

Web site: *www.painconnection.org*

NFP website offers online education and support communities for pain patients and their families, including cancer pain and palliative care resources.

CANCER-PAIN (Association of Cancer Online Resources)

Web page: *www.acor.org Click on "Mailing Lists" and then select "CANCER-PAIN."*

Online discussion list about pain associated with cancer and its treatments.

NCCN Cancer Pain Treatment Guidelines for Patients
Web page: *www.nccn.org/patient_gls/_english/_pain/index.htm*

NCI/PDQ Pain
Web page: *cancer.gov Enter "pain" in the search box.*
Expert-reviewed information summary about cancer-related pain.
Includes discussion of approaches to the management and
treatment of cancer-associated pain.
Abrahm, Janet L. *A Physician's Guide to Pain and Symptom Man-
agement in Cancer Patients.* Baltimore, MD: The Johns Hop-
kins University Press, 2000.
Aimed at health care professionals, this practical and comprehen-
sive textbook is also an excellent resource for patients.

Peripheral Neuropathy

The Neuropathy Association
60 East 42nd Street, Suite 942, New York, NY 10165
Phone: 212–692–0662
Web site: *www.neuropathy.org*

**CANCER-NEUROPATHY (Association of Cancer Online
Resources)**
Web page: *www.acor.org. Click on "Mailing Lists" and then select
"CANCER-NEUROPATHY."*

Print Publications
Online discussion group for patients dealing with neuropathy
induced by cancer or its treatments.

Print Publications
Almadrones, L.A. and R. Arcot. "Patient Guide to Peripheral Neuropathy." *Oncology Nursing Forum* 26, no. 8 (1999): 1359–1362.

Pleural Effusion

**Chemical Pleurodesis for Malignant Pleural Effusion. (Cancer
Supportive Care)**
Web page: *www.cancersupportivecare.com/pleural.html*
Carolyn Clary-Macy, RN, provides a clear explanation of chemical
pleurodesis for malignant pleural effusion. Aimed at patients.

Sexual Effects

CANCER-FERTILITY & CANCER-SEXUALITY (Association of Cancer Online Resources)

Web site: *www.acor.org. Click on "Mailing Lists." and then select "CANCER-FERTILITY" and/or "CANCER-SEXUALITY."*
Online discussion lists about fertility and sexuality issues associated with cancer.

NCI/PDQ Sexuality and Reproductive Issues

Web page: *cancer.gov Enter "sexuality" in the search box.*
Expert-reviewed information summary about factors that may affect fertility and sexual functioning in people who have cancer.

Tests & Procedures

Diagnostic Imaging (MEDLINEplus)

Web page: *www.nlm.nih.gov/medlineplus/diagnosticimaging.html*

Laboratory Tests (MEDLINEplus)

Web page: *www.nlm.nih.gov/medlineplus/laboratorytests.html*

Print Publications

Margolis, Simeon, ed. *The Johns Hopkins Consumer Guide to Medical Tests: What You Can Expect, How You Should Prepare, What Your Results Mean.* Baltimore, MD: The Johns Hopkins University Press, 2001.

Treatment Information & Guidelines

NCCN Lung Cancer Treatment Guidelines for Patients

Web page: *www.nccn.org/patient_gls/_english/_lung/index.htm*

NCI/PDQ Non-small Cell Lung Cancer Treatment & Small Cell Lung Cancer Treatment

Web page: *cancer.gov Enter "lung cancer" in the search box and then select "Lung Cancer Home Page."*
Expert-reviewed summaries about the treatment of NSCLC and SCLC.

Chemotherapy and You (NIH/NCI)
Web page: *cancer.gov Enter "Chemotherapy and You" in the search box. Also available in print by calling 800–4CANCER.*

Radiation Therapy and You (NIH/NCI)
Web page: *cancer.gov Enter "Radiation Therapy and You" in the search box. Also available in print by calling 800–4CANCER.*

Your Surgery
Web site: *www.yoursurgery.com Select "Chest" and then "Thoracotomy."*
Detailed explanation of thoracotomy, including discussion of lobectomy and pneumonectomy.

Print Publications
McKay, Judith and Nancee Hirano. *The Chemotherapy and Radiation Therapy Survival Guide.* Oakland, CA: New Harbinger Publications, Inc., 1998.
Olson, Kaye. *Surgery and Recovery.* Traverse City, MI: Rhodes & Easton, 1998.

Survivorship Issues
LT-SURVIVORS (Association of Cancer Online Resources)
Web page: *www.acor.org Click on "Mailing Lists" and then select "LT-SURVIVORS."*
Forum for discussion of issues of concern to long-term cancer survivors.

Print Publications
Harpham, Wendy Schlessel. *After Cancer: A Guide to Your New Life.* New York: W.W. Norton & Company, 1994.

Women and Minorities
National Women's Health Information Center
8550 Arlington Boulevard, Suite 300, Fairfax, VA 22031
Phone: 800–994–9662
Web site: *www.4women.gov*

Office of Minority Health
P.O. Box 37337, Washington, DC 20013–7337
Phone: 800–444–6472
Web site: *www.omhrc.gov*

Appendix

Glossary

Adenocarcinoma: a type of non-small cell lung cancer; a malignant tumor that arises from glandular tissue

Adjuvant therapy: therapy given after initial treatment to increase its effectiveness; for example, adjuvant chemotherapy following surgery

Advanced directives: legal documents that allow you to prepare for future medical possibilities and to assign someone to act on your behalf in the event you become unable to direct your own medical care

Alopecia: hair loss

Alveoli: tiny air sacs that compose the lungs

Anemia: low red blood cell count; may cause tiredness, weakness, and shortness of breath

Angiogenesis: the formation of new blood vessels that allows tumors to grow

Angiogenesis inhibitors: drugs that prevent the formation of new blood vessels

Anti-emetics: drugs that prevent nausea and vomiting

Apoptosis: process by which normal cells die; often referred to as "programmed cell death"

Asymptomatic: without symptoms

Benign: not cancerous; not life-threatening

Biopsy: removal of tissue or fluid sample for microscopic examination

Bone scan: an imaging test in which a radionuclear substance is injected into the veins and taken up by the bones in areas of potential metastatic disease

Brachytherapy: internal radiation therapy that involves placing "seeds" of radioactive material near or in the tumor

Bronchioloalveolar carcinoma (BAC): a type of adenocarcinoma

Bronchoscope: see **Bronchoscopy**

Bronchoscopy: a procedure that involves inserting a flexible tube (bronchoscope) through the nose down into the lungs. Needles can be inserted through the bronchoscope to obtain biopsy samples.

Carcinogens: cancer-causing substances

Carcinogenesis: the development of cancer

Cells: microscopic units that make up the organs of the body

Centigray: unit of radiation

Central venous catheter (CVC): a thin tube that is surgically inserted to allow access to large veins

Chemoprevention: the use of natural or synthetic substances to prevent cancer

Chemopreventive agent: a natural or synthetic substance used to prevent cancer

Chemotherapy: the use of medicine to treat cancer

Chromosomes: strands of DNA and proteins in cell nucleus that carry units of heredity (genes)

Chronic obstructive pulmonary disease (COPD): chronic bronchitis or emphysema

Clinical trials: research studies involving people

Clubbing: a condition that causes the nails on the fingers to bulge out; clubbing occurs with many different types of lung problems

Colony stimulating factors: substances that stimulate bone marrow to increase production of blood cells; also referred to as growth factors

Complete blood count (CBC): a blood test that details the quantities of white blood cells, red blood cells, and platelets

COX-2 inhibitors: substances that inhibit production of proteins called prostaglandins

CT scan (computed tomography): computerized series of x-rays that create a detailed cross-sectional image of the body

Deep vein thrombosis (DVT): a blood clot occurring in a deep-lying vein in the leg or pelvis

Differentiation: a term used to describe the degree to which tumor tissue resembles normal tissue

DNA (deoxyribonucleic acid): the "brains" of a cell; DNA is composed of chromosomes

Electrolytes: acids, bases, and salts essential for maintaining life; electrolyte abnormalities are imbalances of salts or chemicals in the blood

Esophagus: the tube through which food travels from the mouth to the stomach

Fibrosis: scarring of the lung

First-line therapy: initial treatment

Fraction: single treatment of radiation; a radiation dose is divided into fractions

Gene: unit of heredity that regulates a particular function; located on a specific place on a chromosome

Gene therapy: treatment that replaces the abnormal gene in a cancer cell with a normal gene

Grade: term used to describe the degree to which tumor tissue resembles normal tissue

Growth factors: substances that stimulate cells to grow; drugs that help the bone marrow recover from the effects of chemotherapy (see also **colony-stimulating factors**)

Gray (Gy): modern unit of radiation dosage (older unit is a rad)

Growth factor inhibitors: substances that inhibit the growth factors that stimulate cells to grow

Hilar lymph nodes: lymph nodes located in the region where the bronchus meets the lung

Histology/histological: tissue type; assessment of cellular features by microscopic evaluation

Hospice: a concept of end-of-life care that focuses on palliative rather than curative care and provides comprehensive support to dying patients and their families

Incidence: the number of new cases of a cancer (or any disease or event) in a defined population during a set period of time

Informed consent: a process that provides potential participants in a clinical trial the information they need to make an informed decision about whether or not to participate

Intensity Modulated Radiation Therapy (IMRT): a type of three-dimensional radiation therapy (3D-CRT) that uses radiation beams of varying strengths

Interventional radiologist: a radiologist who uses x-rays and other imaging techniques to perform minimally invasive medical procedures

Intravenous: in the vein

Large cell carcinoma: a type of non-small cell lung cancer

Lobectomy: surgical removal of a lobe of the lung

Lymph node: small collections of white blood cells scattered throughout the body

Lymph node dissection: surgical removal of lymph nodes

Lymphatic system: a vascular system that contains lymph nodes; cancer can spread through the lymphatic system.

Main stem bronchi: the two main breathing tubes (right main stem bronchus and left main stem bronchus) that branch off the trachea

Main stem bronchus: see **Main stem bronchi**

Malignant: cancerous; cells that exhibit rapid, uncontrolled growth and can spread to other parts of the body

Mediastinal lymph nodes: lymph nodes located in the mediastinum, the area between the lungs.

Mediastinoscopy: a surgical procedure by which lymph nodes can be removed for microscopic examination

Medical oncologist: a physician who performs comprehensive management of cancer patients throughout all phases of care; specializes in treating cancer with medicine

Metastasis: the spread of cancer from the initial cancer site to other parts of the body

Mini-thoracotomy: a type of minimally invasive chest surgery

Mutation: a damaged gene

Nadir: lowest measured value; period of low blood counts

Negative margins: a phrase used when normal tissue is found at the edge of the biopsy sample

Neoadjuvant therapy: therapy given before the primary therapy; for example, neoadjuvant chemotherapy, which is sometimes given prior to surgery

Neovascularization: formation of new blood vessels that allows tumors to grow

Neuropathy: see **Peripheral neuropathy**

Neutropenia: low white blood cell count

Neutrophil: a type of white blood cell that attacks bacteria

Nicotine replacement therapy: smoking cessation method that uses nicotine substitutes in various forms, including a patch, gum, inhaler, or nasal spray

Non-small cell lung cancer (NSCLC): a type of lung cancer that includes adenocarcinoma, squamous cell carcinoma, and large cell carcinoma

Oncogene: a mutated gene that can allow a cell to grow uncontrollably

Oncology nurse: a specialized nurse trained to provide care to cancer patients

Oncology social worker: a social worker trained to provide counseling and practical assistance to cancer patients.

Palliative care specialist: a physician trained in pain management

Palliation: see **Palliative treatment**

Palliative treatment: treatment given not with the intent to cure but with the intent to prolong survival and reduce symptoms from the tumor

Pancoast tumor (superior sulcus tumor): a tumor occurring near the top of the lungs that may cause shoulder pain or weakness, or a group of symptoms including a droopy eyelid, dry eyes, and lack of sweating on the face

Paraneoplastic symptoms: symptoms that result from substances released by cancer cells and that occur at a site not directly involved with the tumor

Parietal pleura: a membrane lining the chest wall

Passive smoking: inhaling secondhand smoke

Pathologist: a physician trained to examine and evaluate cells and tissue.

Patient controlled analgesia (PCA): a method by which a patient can regulate the amount of pain medication he or she receives

Performance status: the general condition of the patient

Pericardial effusion: accumulation of fluid inside the sac (pericardium) that surrounds the heart

Peripheral neuropathy: tingling, numbness, or burning sensation in hands, feet, or legs caused by damage to peripheral nerves by a tumor or by chemotherapy or radiation

PET scan (positron emission tomography): a nuclear medicine imaging test that measures metabolism; can differentiate between healthy and abnormal tissue

Phlebotomist: a technician trained to draw blood

Photodynamic therapy (PDT): treatment that uses laser light to kill cancer cells

Placebo: an inactive substance

Platelet: a type of blood cell responsible for clotting

Pleura: a membrane surrounding the lung (visceral pleura) and lining the chest wall (parietal pleura)

Pleural effusion: accumulation of fluid between the outside of the lung and the inside of the chest wall

Pleural space: the area between the outside of the lung and the inside of the chest wall

Pleurodesis: a procedure to prevent recurrence of pleural effusion by draining the fluid and inserting medication into the pleural space

Pneumonectomy: surgical removal of the entire lung

Pneumonia: an inflammatory infection of the lung

Pneumonitis: irritation of the lungs

Port: a type of central venous catheter that is surgically implanted under the skin

Positive margins: a phrase used when cancer cells are found at the edge of the biopsy sample

Prognosis: predicted outcome; likelihood of survival

Prophylactic cranial irradiation (PCI): radiation to the brain with the intention of preventing the development of brain metastases

Pulmonary embolism (PE): a blood clot that travels to the lungs causing full or partial blockage of one or both pulmonary arteries

Pulmonary function tests (PFTs): a group of breathing tests used to determine lung health

Pulmonologist: a physician who specializes in the diagnosis and treatment of lung diseases

Rad: unit of radiation

Radiation fibrosis: scarring of the lungs caused by radiation treatment

Radiation oncologist: a physician who specializes in treating cancer with radiation

Radiation therapy: treatment that uses high-dose x-rays or other high energy rays to kill cancer cells

Radiofrequency ablation (RFA): treatment that uses high-frequency electric current to kill cancer cells

Randomized controlled trial (RCT): a research study in which the participants are assigned by chance (using a computer or a table of random numbers) to separate groups that compare different treatments; a method used to prevent bias in research

Regimen: specific treatment plan; often used in reference to a combination of chemotherapy drugs (type of drug, dosage, and schedule)

Rehabilitation specialist: a person trained to help patients recover from physical changes brought about by cancer or cancer treatment

Resectable: able to be surgically removed (resected)

Resection: surgical removal

Respiratory depression: slowing of breathing

Second-line treatment: treatment method(s) used following an initial treatment that either does not stop cancer progression or stops it only temporarily

Small cell carcinoma: a type of lung cancer that differs in appearance and behavior from non-small cell lung cancers (adenocarcinoma, squamous cell carcinoma, large cell carcinoma)

Small cell lung cancer (SCLC): refers to small cell carcinoma, as opposed to non-small cell lung cancers (adenocarcinoma, squamous cell carcinoma, large cell carcinoma)

Sputum: mucous and other secretions produced by the lungs

Squamous cell carcinoma: a type of non-small cell lung cancer

Staging: determining how far cancer has spread

Stent: a hollow tube that can be inserted via bronchoscopy into the airway to prevent it from being blocked or crushed by the tumor

Stereotactic body radiotherapy: a highly precise radiation therapy technique; when used to treat brain metastases, it is called stereotactic radiosurgery

Superior sulcus tumor: see **Pancoast tumor**

Superior vena cava syndrome (SVCS): a collection of symptoms that may include swelling in the neck, shoulders, and arms caused by a lung tumor pressing on the SVC, one of the large vessels leading into the heart

Surgery: removal of tissue by means of an operation (surgical procedure)

Targeted therapy: therapy directed at aspects of the cell that are specific for cancer

Thoracentesis: a procedure that uses a needle to remove fluid from the space between the lung and the chest wall.

Thoracic surgeon: a surgeon who specializes in performing chest surgery

Thoracotomy: a common type of lung surgery that requires a large incision to provide access to the lungs

Three-dimensional radiation therapy (3D-CRT): a type of radiation therapy that enables higher doses of radiation to be delivered more precisely than standard radiation therapy

Thrombocytopenia: low counts of platelets that may result in bruising and/or bleeding

Trachea: breathing tube (airway) leading from the larynx to the lungs

Transthoracic (percutaneous) biopsy: a biopsy obtained by inserting a needle through the skin and chest wall into the tumor

Tumor: a mass of tissue formed by a new growth of cells

Tumor suppressor gene: a gene that can block cancer from developing

Video-assisted Thoracoscopic Surgery (VATS): a type of minimally invasive chest surgery

Visceral pleura: a membrane surrounding the lung

X-ray: high-energy radiation used to image the body

Wedge resection: surgical removal of the tumor and a small amount of lung tissue surrounding the tumor

Index

_____
_____
_____
_____
_____
_____
_____
_____
_____
_____
_____
_____
_____